# Healing the Trauma of Infidelity

Powerful Skills for
Rebuilding Trust and Attachment
to Find Love, Commitment,
and Intimacy Again

William M. Bumberry, PhD

New Harbinger Publications, Inc.

## Publisher's Note

*This publication is designed to provide accurate and authoritative information in regard to the subject matter covered. It is sold with the understanding that the publisher is not engaged in rendering psychological, financial, legal, or other professional services. If expert assistance or counseling is needed, the services of a competent professional should be sought.*

NEW HARBINGER PUBLICATIONS is a registered trademark of New Harbinger Publications, Inc.

New Harbinger Publications is an employee-owned company.

Copyright © 2025 by William Bumberry
New Harbinger Publications, Inc.
5720 Shattuck Avenue
Oakland, CA 94609
www.newharbinger.com

All Rights Reserved

Cover design by Sara Christian

Acquired by Wendy Millstine

Edited by Kandace Little

---

Library of Congress Cataloging-in-Publication Data on file

Printed in the United States of America

| 27 | 26 | 25 | | | | | | | | |
|----|----|----|----|---|---|---|---|---|---|---|
| 10 | 9 | 8 | 7 | 6 | 5 | 4 | 3 | 2 | 1 | First Printing |

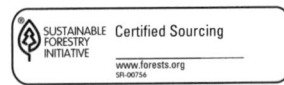

*Dedicated with love to those who are my life…*

*My loving wife, friend, and life partner, Kathy*

*My exquisite daughters, Meg and Laura*

*My rambunctious grandkids, Ben, Tommy, Anna, and Mason*

*And in memory of those who departed too soon but left a legacy of how to live with grace and dignity…*

*My father, William P. Bumberry*

*My mother, Alice A. Bumberry*

*And my beloved sister, Jeanne Jakiela*

# Contents

| | | |
|---|---|---:|
| | Foreword | VII |
| | Acknowledgments | IX |
| | Introduction: Your Darkest Night | 1 |

## Part 1: Regaining Your Balance and Gaining Perspective

| | | |
|---|---|---:|
| CHAPTER 1 | There is a Path | 8 |
| CHAPTER 2 | Understanding Infidelity | 15 |
| CHAPTER 3 | Understanding Relationships: Making Love Last | 26 |

## Part 2: The Decision to Forgive and Communication Skills for the Journey

| | | |
|---|---|---:|
| CHAPTER 4 | The Decision to Forgive | 40 |
| CHAPTER 5 | Essential Communication Skills | 51 |

## Part 3: Healing the Hurt and Building the Bond

| | | |
|---|---|---:|
| CHAPTER 6 | Healing Begins with Atonement | 64 |
| CHAPTER 7 | Attunement: From Avoiding to Addressing Issues | 78 |
| CHAPTER 8 | Attunement: Revitalizing Your Friendship | 98 |
| CHAPTER 9 | The Path to Infidelity | 114 |
| CHAPTER 10 | Attachment: Commitment and Intimacy | 133 |
| CHAPTER 11 | Making It Forever | 152 |
| | References | 159 |

# Foreword

Recovering from infidelity is one of the most profound and painful challenges a couple can face. The breach of trust, the shattering of dreams, and the flood of overwhelming emotions can make the journey seem insurmountable. We have been struck by the struggle they are in and pain couples experience, inspired by their capacity to repair, forgive, and reconnect, and in awe of their ability to rebuild. When the hurt seems too great, ordinary, everyday couples do extraordinary things.

With the right guidance and unwavering support, it is possible not only to survive this crisis but to emerge from it stronger, more resilient, and deeply connected. In this groundbreaking book, Dr. William Bumberry (Bill) provides a clear, compassionate, and effective roadmap for couples seeking to rebuild their relationship after infidelity's devastating blow.

As a Senior Advanced Clinical Gottman Trainer and Consultant, and with decades of experience, Bill has witnessed firsthand the transformative power of the Gottman Method. His deep expertise in the research-based principles developed by Drs. John and Julie Gottman, combined with his distinctive integration of emotion-focused therapy and family systems work, makes him uniquely positioned to guide readers through the complex and often painful process of healing after infidelity.

Within the pages of this book, Bill's warmth, humor, and practical wisdom shine through, offering hope and direction to those who may feel lost or overwhelmed. He skillfully navigates the emotional landscape of betrayal, forgiveness, and the rebuilding of trust, providing couples with the vital tools and strategies they need to heal and reconnect. Whether you are the Hurt Partner, seeking to understand and process your pain, or the Involved Partner, committed to making amends and restoring the relationship, this book will be an invaluable companion on your healing journey.

Bill's professional journey has been shaped by some of the greatest minds in family and couples therapy. Trained, mentored, and befriended by luminaries such as Carl Whitaker, Salvador Minuchin, Sue Johnson, and

John and Julie Gottman, Bill has carved out a distinguished legacy in a field transformed by these legends. His career spans decades of innovation and expertise, and his influence reverberates globally.

As a therapist, mentor, and educator, Bill has profoundly impacted the training of countless relationship therapists worldwide. His dedication to developing skilled clinicians has elevated the standard of care for couples and families everywhere. Through workshops, mentorship, and direct guidance, he has played a pivotal role in shaping a global community of compassionate, competent practitioners.

Bill humbly reflects on his beginnings, often speaking of the invaluable relationships he formed with his mentors. His gratitude for their guidance goes beyond their professional wisdom; it is rooted in the deep, personal connections that shaped his own approach to therapy and life. For Bill, connection is the foundation of all meaningful work—this belief underpins both his clinical practice and his teachings. While he once walked alongside the greats in the field, Dr. William Bumberry is now a towering figure himself—a giant of relationship therapy.

For those of us fortunate enough to walk alongside him, it has been an honor and privilege to share in his journey.

—John Flanagan, AMHSW
partner, Relationship Institute Australasia; principle, Burleigh Heads Psychology and Relationship Clinic

—Trish Purnell-Webb, MPsych(Clin)
partner, Relationship Institute Australasia

# Acknowledgments

Heartfelt thanks to my visionary agent Wendy Millstine, my wise, perceptive, and patient editors Vicraj Gill and Kandace Little, and the team at New Harbinger who made this book possible.

I'd like to express my deepest appreciation to John and Julie Gottman for doing the research and creating the clinical model that is at the core of this book. Their lifelong dedication to couples has changed the landscape of dealing with the trauma of betrayal. They've developed skills and created exercises that bring healing to places of pain that were previously inaccessible. This model has also changed the way therapists around the globe work with the trauma of infidelity. My first encounter with their Trust Revival Method was in *What Makes Love Last?* (Gottman and Silver 2012). In the years that followed, they refined the model and created a training program for therapists entitled "Treating Affairs and Trauma: Helping Couples Heal and Rebuild Trust" (Gottman and Gottman 2017). This model is central to my clinical work as well as much of the material found in this book. Heartfelt thanks to John and Julie Gottman for granting permission for the use of this material. On a more personal note, I'd like to thank John and Julie for decades of inspiration, support, and friendship. It's been and remains a privilege.

Additional thanks to my extraordinary colleagues and friends in the Gottman community. Ideas formed from decades of collaboration with Vagdevi Meunier, John Flanagan, Trish Purnell-Webb, Don Cole, Carrie Cole, Kim Panganiban, Lynda Voorhees Davis, Don Allen, Chris Cambas, and Dave Penner have found their way into my writing. I'd also like to thank the dedicated women and men who are the Gottman Institute.

Most importantly, love and appreciation to Kathy, my wife, life partner, and inspiration for more than fifty years. Life brightened the day we met. She taught me that a lifetime of love is possible. I've been blessed to walk the path with her. My bright, loving, compassion-filled daughters, Laura and Meghan, have added depth and joy to life since the day of their arrival.

I'm so impressed by and proud of them. They're my greatest contribution to our planet. They taught me how to be a dad and continue to do so. Their joyous, energetic, life-filled kids, my grandkids Ben, Tommy, Anna, and Mason, add another level of depth to life. They're teaching me the intricacies of grandparenting.

INTRODUCTION

# Your Darkest Night

Betrayal is our greatest fear…our darkest night. And now it's arrived at your door and entered your life. Not invited, not deserved, but it's here. Your partner has crossed the line into infidelity and is involved with another person.

You no longer have the option of avoiding this fear. You can't deny it. You can't go back in time and change the course of history. It's happened. Perhaps it's still happening. How can you know for sure? You're devastated, angry, scared. It's difficult to think clearly. Hard to see a way through the turmoil. You're not sure there's a path to save your relationship. Is that even what you want?

This book is a guide to help you weather the storm, regain your balance, and work through a process to help you decide on your future.

You've lived years, perhaps decades, in a committed relationship with your partner. You've been through so much together. You've experienced wonderful times together. Close and connected. Intense and passionate. There was no place you would rather be. No one else you wanted to be with. You were sure of the depth of your relationship, the strength of your bond. Was it always easy? Of course not. Relationships involve ups and downs. Joys and pain. At times, it was really difficult, but you hung in there and worked it out with your partner.

And now your life is in pieces. Your relationship shattered. Your inner world in disarray. You might even wonder, *Was our relationship real? Was it ever real? Was I deluding myself?* Questions that were unthinkable now flood into your consciousness. You're trying to make sense of the impossible. The foundation of your life now lies in shambles at your feet.

## Understanding Your Trauma

Just so you know, your reactions are not unusual. They're not signs of weakness, neediness, or codependency. They're not to be misconstrued as evidence of immaturity. They're about trauma. A primordial dread of abandonment resides within each of us. It's what it means to be human. You're not designed to be alone. Can you survive alone? Sure. But at your core, you're created for connection. Not superficial, convenient connection but personal, engaged, intimate connection. Difficult times, even tragedies, are eased when shared with others…with connected others. People you can turn to and rely on—with trusted others.

This is what makes the betrayal of infidelity such a devastating type of abandonment. The loss of trust. The *shattering* of trust. What was real becomes illusory. The promises and agreements you made and committed to have been changed. Not changed by a conversation, or even an "out in the open" fight, but rather by a secretive, unilateral decision. You had no voice in a decision that altered the fabric and flow of your life.

And it's about more than not having a voice or suffering a unilateral change; it's also about being replaced. Your partner not only moved away from you, but they moved toward someone else. The emotional honesty and physical exclusivity you pledged to one another have been violated.

## Perspective on Infidelity

It's important to note that you are not alone. The lifetime rates of infidelity indicate that 20–40 percent of couples experience the crisis of infidelity in their relationships (Atkins et al., 2001; Peluso 2019; Irvine 2022). The aftermath of this type of betrayal is life changing and relationship altering. There's nothing good about it. If you could go back to the time before the betrayal, you would. I wish you could. But there's no way to "unring the bell." The challenge here is to decide what you're going to do with it: how you'll handle the storm, deal with the trauma, and decide on your future.

As you try to make sense of your partner's infidelity, it's important to realize there's a lot of information out there. Some valid, other information…not so much. What infidelity is and what it isn't! What it says about you. What it means about your partner. Does it mean you have a bad relationship? Is it your fault? Is it inevitable? Is there hope? The questions are endless. How do you handle and process all the information coming your way?

One thing that seems quite clear is that, once infidelity enters your relationship, you'll see it everywhere. Suddenly the news, your social media, what you hear about friends, neighbors, movie stars, and politicians, are full of infidelity. Movies you watch, television series you bring into your home, sitcoms, and even comedians all seem focused on infidelity and betrayal. This is to be expected. It's become personal to you. It leaps from the screen, from your phone, and into your psyche. It's everywhere. You can't get away from it.

So, step one is to slow down and balance yourself.

Your task begins with recognizing that while infidelity is common, and you now notice it around every corner, the betrayal of infidelity in your life is also specific to your unique relationship. Comparing your relationship to others is risky.

Here are a few points to begin with:

You did not cause your partner to cheat!

Your partner's infidelity does not necessarily mean they don't value and love you.

Infidelity does not necessarily mean you have a bad relationship.

Infidelity doesn't mean you can never be close, intimate, and happy together again.

Infidelity doesn't mean your relationship is hopeless or over.

But it does mean that you have work to do! You have issues to face and decisions to make. The advice, opinions, and perspectives of others may be of value to you at times. At other times they won't serve you well; they're exactly what you *don't* need. It's a time for wisdom, patience and balance.

As you read the chapters and work through the exercises, remember that the intent is to help you make the right decision about your future. There may be times when you feel hopeful, only to be followed by moments when it's just too much. The hope is that after you've done the work, you'll have clarity about your path.

## What's Next

This book is a guide to help you address and deal with the trauma of your partner's infidelity. It's a time for healing, soul searching, focus, and clarity of thought. It's a time to center yourself, strengthen yourself, and work through the devastation of the moment with an eye toward your future. What are your options? Do you see a path? What would you like to happen? What's possible?

This book is also a guide designed to help you work with your partner to restore trust and rebuild your bond. The ideas and exercises you encounter can be the basis for creating a healthy, connected, sustainable relationship. When working on the exercises, please write your responses in a journal. This will be an important resource as you move forward. Worksheets based on the exercises within the book are also available online.

In most cases, this new relationship is more than just re-creating what you had before the betrayal. There are unaddressed issues to face. There are communication skills and relationship muscles to develop. It's not just about staying together or not divorcing. It's about creating a connection that's more personal and intimate. The journey requires courage and commitment. While at times daunting, it's doable. There is hope!

The clinical model presented here is based on and adapted from the work of John and Julie Gottman. The Gottman Trust Revival Method introduced the paradigm-shifting Atone-Attune-Attach approach to recovering from the trauma of infidelity (Gottman and Gottman 2017).

## Who This Book Is For

Infidelity is a painful, disorienting, and life-changing experience. There's no simple solution to it or easy path through it. But there is hope! This book is designed to help you, the Hurt Partner (HP), regain your balance and see if you want to try to move forward together. To decide if you want to work with your partner to not only heal the hurt but also endeavor to create a healthy, sustainable, loving relationship out of the loss and chaos you're experiencing. If the time is right, and this is the direction you choose, you and your partner will then be guided through a process to create a path to that destination.

If your partner is interested in joining you to create that healthy, sustainable, loving relationship, this book will be of interest and value to them too. They'll come away with a deeper understanding of what you're going through and what it will take to heal and move to a more connected future together. Sections of the book are written directly for them. They'll be invited, and challenged, to take responsibility for the pain they caused as well as for creating the conditions for healing.

The third section of the book focuses on you and your partner working together to repair and rebuild what has been damaged or destroyed.

But first a word of caution. This book is not a substitute for therapy with a professional therapist trained to work with the trauma of betrayal. For many of you, it may offer what you need to reengage and begin the healing journey. For others, it may serve as a useful adjunct to therapy. Throughout this volume, you'll work on many of the themes and issues the pain of betrayal evokes. Some will resonate with you more than others. At all times, exercise your own judgment regarding what works for you. Don't push yourself into areas you're not ready to enter.

# Part 1

# Regaining Your Balance and Gaining Perspective

This section is primarily for you, the Hurt Partner (HP). It's a working section for you to look at the situation and clarify your position about the path ahead. Chapter 2 offers an understanding of infidelity, while Chapter 3 describes essential components of healthy relationships. You're asked to explore your position and assess the quality of your relationship. Even though most of it is directed to you, your partner will benefit from reading this section.

CHAPTER 1

# There is a Path

These are difficult times! Your world is shattered. You've lost your center. Disoriented and confused, you're at a loss about what to do next, how to even manage the day, and regain your inner balance.

The discovery that your partner is having an affair cracked the foundation of your relationship and the walls came tumbling down. Trust is impossible and commitment is but a hollow word. Your thoughts of the future (*what future?*) are a roiling, chaotic, confusing swirl. Everything you built, the work of a lifetime, everything you believed in, all that you dedicated your life to is gone in a flash...or so it seems. There's no way to rationalize or sugarcoat this moment: you're at a crossroad. Not one of your own choosing, but a crossroad nonetheless.

You're in a season of strong emotions and crucial decisions. Whether you blow up or shut down, move toward or move away. Whether you give voice to your rage or anguish or fear, or the blend of emotions the betrayal has evoked, feelings bubble. It's a time of deep emotions and intense reactivity. It's also a time of *mixed* emotions. Emotions travel in clusters. When anger opens and rage follows, you may attack and blame. Even in the midst of a "rage moment," fear and anguish, sadness and worry are but a step away. They too will have their time. They too clammer for expression.

In the disorientation, terror, rage, and hopelessness of the moment, the trauma of the moment, it may be impossible to look forward and see a path. Not a broken path of just staying together, hobbling along and "tolerating the intolerable," but a path of true connection and joy. It's hard to imagine that your relationship could ever feel right again. And there is some truth to those feelings. Something has irrevocably changed. That bone-deep sense of trust, the "knowing" that "you would never betray me," that "*you could never* betray me" is gone ... forever. This isn't an issue of you refusing to "move on" or "let it go." It's not a function of you not forgiving. The betrayal is real; it actually happened. It's an experience, not a fear or worry. It resides in your nervous system. It's stored in your brain. It's now part of your lived experience, part of your history. You'll never forget it.

And yet there is hope. There is a path to walk. Or more accurately, there is a path to create. A path to cut into the forest of confusion, fear, hopelessness, and uncertainty that engulfs you. I'm not suggesting it's easy, but I am suggesting it's possible to face this crisis with courage and dignity. To traverse the course with the kind of integrity that will allow you to feel whole again. Although you didn't ask for it, there is a journey in front of you. It may be one you've feared all your life. Perhaps it's one you never even considered. But like it or not, it's here. The truth is it's already underway. You're already in the early phases of choosing a path, of creating your future.

In this chapter, you'll begin that journey. You'll look at your situation and consider the path forward. You'll decide if repair is something you wish to pursue.

## Calming the Storm

While you have a journey to take and decisions to make, you're not traveling alone. Your partner also has a journey to take and decisions to make. It's a time for soul searching and prioritizing—for both of you. At one level, it's a time for exploring your wants, wishes, and needs. At another, it's about going deeper, visiting your values and deciding if they will be your guide.

But above all else, at the beginning of this journey, it's about calming the storm and establishing safety. Part of this is a study in self-regulation. Of learning to slow down and settle yourself in a time of overwhelming fear and agonizing loneliness. Anger and anxiety, confusion, and a lack of clarity leave you feeling vulnerable. At times, helpless. Moments of tenuous hopefulness are too easily shattered.

Getting through the storm is not a one-person process. We're created for connection and closeness. Our hearts long for it. Our nervous systems need it. Yes, you can create distance as you try to minimize risk. And at times that may be the wise thing to do, at least temporarily. But in the long run, distance as a primary relationship strategy guarantees the very thing you dread the most: loneliness. Remember, we're created for connection.

And, protect yourself you must. You're still wounded, bleeding. To truly stop the pain, you need the presence of a caring, compassionate other. Family and friends can be of great benefit in these moments. They can be indispensable. You need safety and security. But be careful of who you let in. This is not a time for naïve or foolish trust.

In the best of all worlds, some of the caring and support, the compassion, connection, and closeness you "need" will come from your partner. You're here because you have some hope, or feel some possibility, that the person who betrayed you can still be that supportive, loving partner. The person you chose to share your life with, walk the path with, grow old with, may be the person with the most potential to help resurrect the dream that once compelled you. But are they "safe"? Can you count on them? They've turned away from you. They've betrayed you and the commitments they made to you. If they've done it once, they could do it again. That's a lot to ask your nervous system to overlook. It's a lot to ask of yourself.

You have a role; your partner has a role. But, of course, it's not quite that easy. You're in the challenging position of both strengthening yourself and allowing the very person who wounded you to be part of the solution. We naturally flinch and step back from that kind of vulnerability. We're wired to protect ourselves from danger, not put ourselves at risk.

While we all "know" that to be in a relationship involves some degree of vulnerability, we also often believe our love is different. Betrayals happen to other people, not people like us. Our love is special. "Special," yes; bulletproof, no. So, in the face of the devastating pain of betrayal, how do we decide once again to risk and reach out?

This brings us to the crucial issue of trust. True trust, the inner experience of trust, is something earned, not given. You can try to trust someone. You can say you trust someone. But your body and nervous system do their own calculations. Deep inside, you either feel trusting or you don't. It's based on experience, not wishful thinking. This is not to say that trust, once broken, can never be reestablished. Just that it's not a given. It's not automatic. And in cases of deep betrayal, the passage of time isn't enough. To a large extent, the rebuilding of trust will be the compass that guides your journey. Trust is an essential ingredient for sustainable, intimate relationships.

> *So let me offer a few words to you, the Involved Partner (IP):*
>
> You too have much to face. Right out of the box, one crucial issue to explore is your willingness to own your actions and face their impact. Do you feel remorse for your actions and the pain they caused? And is it real remorse, felt from within? Or are you checking boxes, doing what you think you should do, or saying what your partner needs to hear so they will "get over it"? Another task is to notice if you are experiencing a growing feeling of compassion for your partner and their hurt. These initial reflections end up being essential components of the healing process.
>
> And, to be fair, of course you have reasons for doing what you did. Many people who turn to others are experiencing some degree of sadness, frustration, and above all, loneliness in their relationship. Yes, you may have your own pain. It's real and needs to be addressed. But that pain, those reasons, aren't justifications for *deciding* to engage in the betrayal of having an affair.
>
> I emphasize the word "deciding" intentionally. The truth is that you always have choices. Even here, you had a choice. You had other options. Even now, as you read and reflect on these words, you have options. You can take them in and begin to face what they say about you. You can step up to how infidelity has affected your partner, or you can allow your *rebuttal brain* to make the case for why it's different in your situation: the kind of justification that commonly accompanies betrayal.
>
> Yes, your brain is creative in coming up with reasons and convincing you that, in this case, whatever you did is understandable. But being *understandable* doesn't make it *right*. Sometimes the reasons seem obvious. At other times, they're deep, complex, and difficult to see, let alone admit. The work of facing yourself, probing your depths, and honestly exploring your decision to move into betrayal is an important part of the healing process.

> While the recovery journey takes place over time, it begins with admitting you were wrong and feeling remorse for your actions. It also involves seeing the depth of your partner's pain and dedicating yourself to making amends.
>
> Keep in mind, you're not defined by your mistakes. It's the courage, conviction, and compassion your mistakes awaken that become your measure.

## Is Repair the Right Path?

So take a step back to consider if doing the work and walking this path—toward relationship repair—is right for you. It's a decision you and your partner need to take time to consider. It's not a given. You don't *need* to do this, but to do it, you must *decide* to do it.

The good news is that there is a way to face this difficult time, a way to heal the hurt and establish trust, and learn to connect and communicate as you move toward a more loving relationship.

### Exercise: Is Repair Right for Me?

*This exercise is for you, the HP.*

Consider the following questions. Please write your responses in a journal.

1. Given all you've been through, the pain you've experienced: if this relationship *could* feel right again, is it the one you would choose?

2. Are you sure? Are you ambivalent…sometimes yes, sometimes no?

3. What are your primary reasons for staying? Take a few minutes to list them.

4. Even if you're sure you want to make your relationship work, you likely have some doubts or fears. Take a few minutes to list those fears and doubts too.

5. With trust broken it's hard to know how to get it back. You might wonder, *I don't know if I can ever trust them again. Can I let them back in? Am I willing to try? Am I ready to try?"* What do you need to feel safe enough to begin to trust your partner again? Take a moment to list some of these needs.

### Exercise: Can I Walk This Path?

*This exercise is for the IP.*

While you too may have some relationship concerns, there's a fundamental difference here...you're the person who had the affair. Do you accept the idea that, in the beginning, much of the responsibility to stabilize the relationship is on you? Here are a few questions to start with:

1. Have you ended the affair? If not, are you willing to end it? What can you do to prove this to your partner?

2. Are you willing to do the work required to help your partner feel safe? Will you offer the transparency and confirmation of truth your partner needs?

3. Are you *willing* to commit to your partner?

4. Are you *ready* to begin that work of committing to your partner?

5. Given all you've been through, do you want to stay in this relationship? Are you sure? Are you ambivalent...sometimes yes, sometimes no? Take a few minutes to list your primary reasons for staying.

> 6. Even if you're sure you want to make your relationship work, you may have some doubts or fears. Take a few minutes to list your primary doubts and fears about staying.

## Gathering Your Thoughts

Addressing these questions is a challenging task. They require you to slow down and focus on your pain as well the possibilities. On hope, as well as fear. So, take a moment and a breath. These are complicated issues. While you may lean in one direction, you may be pulled in another at the same time. This is normal! Ambivalence and uncertainty are common reactions to relationship pain. While you desperately want the solace and security of connection, you also fear the devastation of even more hurt. If the relationship didn't mean that much to you, you could simply walk away. But if what you had was real, leaving isn't so easy.

So put your journal down and be kind to yourself. Take a walk, immerse yourself in nature. Call a friend or family member. Meditate, pray, turn to your religious or spiritual practices. Give yourself a break. After a bit of time has passed, when you're feeling rested, perhaps even refreshed, revisit the questions. Notice what you would add to your responses, what you would change. These are living, fluid answers. They evolve over time. During periods of stress, they may even change moment to moment. But for now, take that break so you can gather your thoughts.

## Closing Comments

This chapter is the beginning of your journey. You've started the process of facing your pain and considering the future. You're acknowledging the fact that amid the chaos and devastation you experience, you must decide how to move forward. The torrent of emotions inside you need expression and soothing. This is not the time for the final decision about your relationship. It's the time for the initial decision that you are willing and ready to do the work required to reach clarity.

In the next step, we will take a deeper look at infidelity.

CHAPTER 2

# Understanding Infidelity

The foundation of your relationship relies on how connected and secure you feel with your partner. Because of this, it's no surprise that your partner's betrayal is one of the most distressing experiences of your life. To be truthful, it's more than distressing—it's disorienting. It turns life upside down. While betrayal comes in many shapes and sizes, infidelity, with the dual components of emotional and sexual betrayal, ranks near the top of the pain index.

It's not a stretch to call what you're experiencing traumatic. This trauma has profound implications not only for your initial reaction to the discovery of your partner's affair but also, perhaps more importantly, for the healing. While the foundation of your emotional bond can be destroyed in a flash, the healing that follows takes time.

In the wake of the discovery of the affair, you may experience classic PTSD symptoms such as intrusive thoughts, flashbacks, hypervigilance, or sleep disturbance. These are not signs of you being overemotional, childish, or immature. They're indicators of the panic and trauma that follow betrayal. This becomes a "double betrayal," making it even more painful if your partner denies it or directly lies to you.

To the extent that your partner's denial seemed sincere, to the degree their words were convincing, the wound is even deeper, the path to recovery steeper. It's even more complex if your partner, in the midst of denial, accuses you of being crazy, controlling, or paranoid. Worse yet, they blame you for their actions. Now, in addition to dealing with the original betrayal, you're left with the realization that under duress, your partner might sacrifice your emotional well-being to save themselves. Trust shatters.

Another level of complexity in intimate relationship betrayal is that the person who caused the injury—your partner—is the same person you need to lead the healing process. While the path is not insurmountable, it is steep and full of obstacles. To begin, your partner must accept full responsibility for the affair and acknowledge how deeply it damaged you. They must also feel and express genuine remorse for their actions. It is only from this place that you can begin to move toward healing. Their ability to accept responsibility and express heartfelt remorse offers hope and provides the motivation to even begin the healing journey.

This is not to say that your partner may not have their own hurt, their own pain. They typically have reasons for going down the path of betrayal. And yet, they always had other choices. Becoming involved with another person was not their only option. Addressing this part of the equation is also essential to the ultimate rebuilding of the bond.

Let's now direct our attention to understanding infidelity and exploring your responsibility as well as your partner's. We'll explore how justification blocks healing, how forgiveness is much more than a simple restart, and how vulnerability is essential to authentic connection.

# Defining Infidelity

What constitutes infidelity may seem obvious, and in some cases it is. In others it can be an elusive term to define. But having a clear, shared definition is an important starting point. Is infidelity a moral issue about *right* or *wrong*? Is it an ethical consideration reflecting your community's standard? Do you view it through a spiritual, religious, or a practical lens? Is it an individual "right" or a relationship violation? There are many ways to look at it…all worthy of conversation.

Here's the definition I would encourage you to consider: infidelity is (1) the breaking of an explicit or implicit understanding between partners regarding emotional and/or physical intimacy that is then (2) kept secret when this understanding is violated.

On the surface, this sounds simple. What you consider a violation of your understanding with your partner seems obvious. It's embedded in assumptions about monogamy, trust, commitment, honesty, and personal integrity. While it's impossible to make a comprehensive list of "rules" that cover every situation, the line seems clear. This line is what made the violation so shocking. The idea that it was violated and then kept secret confirms the notion that your partner knew they were crossing the line.

Let's start by exploring your position on infidelity and the understanding between you and your partner. As painful as this can be, it's an important step.

> ### Exercise: **Understanding Your Understanding**
>
> *This exercise is for the HP.*
>
> - What was the nature of the infidelity? What do you believe happened?
>   - Was it primarily physical?
>   - Was it primarily emotional?
>   - Was it both?
> - Describe your version of your understanding or agreement with your partner.
>   - Describe how it was violated. Where was the line crossed?
> - How was it kept secret? Was it hidden, lied about, denied?
>   - Even if your partner admitted or confessed the infidelity…were parts still kept secret?
> - Did your partner blame you?

Okay, this was a difficult exercise. It likely opened some raw feelings. Take a break, take care of yourself.

## Accepting Responsibility vs. Self-Justification

You may be the best partner on the planet. Or you may be like the rest of us; you have flaws, quirks, and moments you're not proud of. You may have said things better left unsaid or done things better not done. Perhaps at times you have been quick to anger, slow to forgive. You may not always feel like having sex or being affectionate. At times, you're "touched out" and just want to be left alone. You may go through periods when you're moody, down, or withdrawn.

I'm not saying these are your best moments. I am saying they're part of the human condition. And even when you fall into these patterns, just know that your words, actions, moods, and inactions didn't cause your partner to cheat. They may not *like* some of these times, and perhaps that's even understandable, but when it comes down to the decision to cheat, your partner did have other options. You didn't cause them to cheat. They made the decision.

This might sound a bit harsh, but anything short of this level of responsibility leaves you and your partner susceptible to the insidious power of self-justification. When the attempt to explain the "why" of betrayal slides, even a bit, toward justification—if your partner says, "I didn't mean to do it, it was the situation, the alcohol, you were so distant, you refused sex, they came on to me, the temptation was too great"—it undermines the healing process. You need emotional honesty from your partner to begin to settle your shakiness and see a path toward healing.

The concept of *free will* invites us, all of us, to take ownership for what we do and how we conduct our lives. Without it there's no real accountability. The words we say, the things we do, are, in fact, choices we make. Free will doesn't imply good or bad. It's not meant to convey a moral judgement. It's just a way of emphasizing "what is."

Does your partner accept responsibility for what they did? Are they holding themselves accountable? Or are they lapsing into self-justification —seeking an explanation for the infidelity that lets them off the hook? There are many paths to betrayal. At times it may look as simple as an unexpected opportunity, and at others, alcohol makes the introduction. Conversely, it may be viewed as a right, as "just what men do," or women, or anyone. "It's their nature." We may carry it as a secret, or not-so-secret, principle "to get it as much as you can," or "it's not cheating unless you get caught." Privacy is sometimes invoked to support a "no harm, no foul" mentality. Or perhaps individual rights: "You can't control me."

The vast majority of adults in our culture say they believe infidelity is wrong. And yet, when it comes to them, to *their* relationship, they find reasons to make exceptions. "In my case it's understandable…even justified."

In general, we're not simply impulsive, irrational beings. We have values and beliefs. We have reasons for doing what we do and for not doing what we don't do. But when it comes to matters of the heart or desire, our algorithms may have a bug. We may consider desire a sufficient justification for behaviors that, in the light of day, actually violate who we are. These behaviors wouldn't be acceptable to your partner if *you* made the same choice. These explanations crumble once we pull back the curtain of justification.

What does this all mean to you, the Hurt Partner? It simply means that when your partner continues to justify their actions rather than owning them, they're not yet in a place to be there for you. They can't be honest with you until they're able to be honest with themselves.

## Infidelity Is an Attachment Injury

The pain of infidelity can sometimes be understood as an *attachment injury* (Johnson 2013). That is, a wound that is deep enough, painful enough, that it won't naturally heal with the passage of time. A wound that damaged the very foundation of your relationship. As the HP it's important to evaluate if this description fits how you feel. An attachment injury goes to your core. It may affect how you see yourself. It deeply colors how you see your partner and how you feel about your relationship. It doesn't just bother you, it damages the basic connection you feel with your partner. Trust is broken. You might say, "Never again! I'll never put myself in the position to be hurt like this again." Your confidence in your partner is shattered. You feel you no longer know who they are. "The person I knew would never have done this to me. They couldn't do this to me."

Just to be clear, of course, in the flow of normal relational living there are moments you hurt, disappoint, or frustrate your partner. You may cause them distress or they may lead you to feel upset. You may feel alone, misunderstood, or taken for granted. They may feel lonely. Moments like these are to be expected…at least at times. And if your connection is strong, if you have confidence your partner loves and values you as well as your relationship, these moments may not require major attention. A simple smile or a hug may do. When they have the courage to offer a repair like "Sorry, that was on me. You didn't deserve that" or "I was in a bad mood," it might be enough to return you to a positive place. This is not what I mean when using the term "attachment injury."

Some wounds are like bruises. They heal with little attention. Others are akin to cuts that get infected. They require direct attention. And if the toxins are not treated and removed, they remain in the body doing damage, causing harm. Ignoring them does not heal them. Even if they go dormant, they're still inside you, waiting to open again in times of stress. The betrayal of infidelity isn't a bruise; it's deeper than that. Ignoring this kind of wound and hoping it will go away comes at a cost. It can lead you to feel chronic resentment toward your partner. Vulnerability and intimacy feel risky. Even in periods of calm, there can be a sense of distance. Things just aren't the way they used to be.

The good news is that in many cases, attachment injuries can be healed. The challenge is that it takes courage, conviction, and work. Eventually you'll need to take the risk of again being vulnerable. To put yourself in that position, your partner will first need to truly hear your pain and have a deep sense of compassion for your hurt. They'll also need to take full ownership for their actions and feel genuine remorse.

Let's begin by talking a bit about healing, forgiveness, and vulnerability. Some of the sections that follow are written for you, the Hurt Partner. Some are written for your partner, the Involved Partner.

# Healing

*This is for the IP.*

Your infidelity caused an injury: a broken bond, the loss of trust. The healing must begin there. The emotional presence, caring, and compassion you have for your partner are essential. The capacity to put your own feelings, issues, and needs on the back burner and truly "be there" with your partner is a start. This can't be offered and sustained as a tactic or an act. Can you put your feelings aside and truly focus on your partner? Can you open yourself to hearing, seeing, and feeling their emotions? Can you stay emotionally present as they express their anger, hurt, fear, and hopelessness? Can you allow your partner's pain to touch you, to move you? When you love someone, taking in their pain opens compassion in you. Compassion leads you to feel for them deeply. It also generates the desire to do something to relieve their pain.

Another essential ingredient is remorse. Regardless of your reasons for the affair, no matter how justified you felt, can you recognize and admit that you made a bad choice? You had other options. This doesn't mean the status quo of your relationship was okay, or that you didn't have legitimate complaints. It's just that you could have handled them differently. Genuine remorse has two components: regret for the pain it caused your partner as well as distress because you also betrayed yourself. By crossing the line and then keeping it secret, you may have acted in a manner that violated your own values.

It's from this base that the early phase of recovery flows more smoothly. Your compassion and remorse begin to offer hope for healing the bond. Trust recovery begins with your partner's deep-seated human need for predictability and certainty. With their world shattered, they need something to hang on to. Can you be that something for them? Your emotional presence, openness, and honesty offer a starting point. Working on transparency is the first step. As the IP, you have a decision to make. Are you willing to be transparent? There's no room for more secrecy in this early stage. Your partner needs to know that you're now telling the truth. Not a partial truth but the whole truth. Not just answering questions, although that is part of it, but proactively offering information. No more sins of omission. No more only sharing information if your partner happens to ask the right question. This is a dramatic shift from the avoidance and secrecy that are often part of infidelity.

Transparency is a simple word, but a challenging task. True transparency is an active, even proactive process. You must be dedicated to giving your partner the information they need to heal. They need to know what really happened. To see how it happened. They need the truth, a truth that resonates inside them and begins to feel real to them. They need to feel they're getting the real story.

In addition to uncovering the past, transparency must also be a central part of your future interactions. Are you willing to incorporate transparency, even uncomfortable transparency, into your way of talking with your partner?

For transparency to be a lasting source of real comfort for your partner, something more is required. That something is verification. Verification moves transparency from an act of faith to a belief grounded in information. This may be a challenging position to embrace. It may require you to share, reveal, or "prove" where you were, who you spoke to, or what you did to a degree you've never done before. It may be uncomfortable. This may not be forever, but at least for now it's important.

The specifics of what constitutes verification lies within your partner. What information or access does your partner need in order to feel confident they know the truth? That they're not still being lied to? In the wake of infidelity, trust must be earned, not given. And while it's virtually impossible to prove a negative, that you're *not* doing something, this is part of the challenge. Your partner may ask for access to your devices or freedom to check your phone or bank accounts. Boundaries shift. Things that might have seemed intrusive before the affair now become reasonable. Your openness to helping them heal, to providing what they need to feel more secure, is important. Remember, your attitude matters. Verification offered with patience and compassion hits the mark. When wrapped in resentment, the benefits are minimized.

# Forgiveness

Forgiveness is a complex issue. It's important to begin by recognizing that you don't have to forgive your partner. This is a choice you make. It's your decision. And even if you decide to begin on the path to forgiveness, it's complicated. It's not simply a matter of will power or hitting a reset button. At the intellectual level, you might be able to offer forgiveness. You might be able to say you forgive your partner. And on a certain level that might be true. But as an experience, emotional forgiveness takes time. It will develop in stages based on what happens between you and your partner. In the early part of recovery from infidelity, you may experience the desire to forgive. While there may be a willingness to forgive, it's fragile, tenuous. It can be easily shattered. Over time, with work, your ability to get to forgiveness may increase. You may be able to honestly say, and feel, you have forgiven your partner.

But now, as you begin the journey, are you ready to try to forgive? Does forgiving mean you're able to fully accept what has happened? Does it mean you no longer feel hurt, angry, or resentful? Does it mean your fears are gone? That despair has disappeared? Of course not—this is not how we're wired. At the beginning it may mean that these feeling are less intense, or perhaps you feel them less frequently, but they all still reside within. It's important to remember, that while the betrayal will always be part of your history, it does not have to define your future.

It's also essential to understand that forgiveness is not forgetting. Forgetting betrayal is not something we're programmed to do. We're hardwired to avoid threat and danger. Our memory of danger is one of our most powerful survival tools. It's a survival mechanism deep inside our nervous system. But from where you stand now, you face the question "Is what we once had—what we could have again—worth the risk and the work it will take to get there?"

There are types of forgiveness that are real but that lead you to decide that you're not willing to remain with your partner. That might take the form of redefining the relationship as a friendship or co-parenting relationship. You can forgive and decide to terminate contact with your partner. Or you can forgive and decide to see if the relationship can be restored.

You don't need to make that decision yet. Today, you're making the decision to *try* to forgive. You're stepping onto the field again but with some caution. You may want to trust and believe your partner, but the pain inside you says "beware."

## Vulnerability

A final point to consider is the question of vulnerability. In everyday life you naturally, instinctively, move away from vulnerability. Why expose yourself to hurt, humiliation, or failure if you can avoid it? This leads you to automatically assess risk and act to minimize it. You quickly learn to not put your hand on a hot stove. But in the wake of infidelity, the hot stove is your partner. How can you get close and not be burned again? There is a certain vulnerability you're accepting as you move forward together. The very person you let in, trusted, shared with, leaned on, and were vulnerable with, betrayed you. Your relationship with your partner may be the deepest vulnerability you've experienced. You now feel exposed. The betrayal causes you to question your trust and openness.

At the end of the day, relationships involve risk. Not a naive risk, but the calculated risk of leaning into your partner believing that the potential gains are worth it. It's related to feeling that you can trust your partner again. That they'll not only not betray you again, but that they'll actually *be there for you...with you.*

Part of this decision—to decide whether to be vulnerable again—is a recognition of your own strength. Knowing that, despite the pain, you will survive. You'll be whole again. You'll be able to more forward without them if you need to. That you're choosing to try, not out of need or weakness, but because of the positive potential you see and perhaps the love you once experienced.

## In Closing

There's a lot to consider and absorb. Seeing infidelity as an attachment injury is a call to address rather than avoid addressing it. The path to forgiveness is not direct and the acceptance of vulnerability requires great self-compassion and courage.

For the IP, the challenge of truly accepting responsibility for their actions and owning the impact it has on you is humbling work. Their ability to step up to the call to compassion is crucial. Once they feel true compassion for you, there's a possibility that genuine remorse and transparency will follow.

With the path and challenge more defined, let's now look into the core components of healthy, loving, and sustainable relationships.

CHAPTER 3

# Understanding Relationships: Making Love Last

In the last chapter, you took the time to explore infidelity, a painful but necessary topic if you're to move forward with your eyes wide open. In this chapter, we'll turn the page and take a look at the core elements of loving, lasting relationships. The kind of relationship you'll need if you're going to develop an intimate connection with your partner. We'll start by discussing love, connection, and attachment. We'll then explore the core pillars of trust and commitment, followed by a focus on the relationship between betrayal and loyalty.

## What is Love?

This question has long been the territory of poets and philosophers. Neuroscientists and researchers have now joined the conversation (Lewis, Amini, and Lannon 2000). How would you respond to the age-old question "What is love?"

Is love an emotion or an action…a feeling or a decision?

Is it fleeting or fixed?

Does it come and go, or come and stay?

Is it passion and intensity…or commitment and consistency?

Is it something you fall into or something you build?

Do you suddenly fall out of it…or does it erode over time?

If you lose love, can it be rekindled?

Does it take work, or is it simply there?

Love can be a bit of all of these things. Your life experiences, from birth to who you are today, inform your sense of what love is. This now includes the experience of infidelity. In this chapter, you'll look at what love is by examining three qualities: trust, commitment, and loyalty. We'll examine how these qualities characterized your relationship before the betrayal and how they are manifested in the present.

## The Case for Connection

The quality of your relationships is the quality of your life. And the relationship that has the most powerful impact is the bond that exists between you and your partner. It's a unique relationship in that it can raise you to heights unknown; it can also drop you to depths unimaginable. It can imbue you with a sense of aliveness, well-being, sensuality, and security. It can also leave you broken, lonely, and without hope. It's your earthly experience of heaven or hell. And perhaps you've experienced a bit of both.

Attachment theory, originated by the brilliant John Bowlby, begins with the premise that we're created for connection. Being close and connected to others is not merely something you want or desire…it's something you *need*. Can you exist without close, personal connections? Of course. But to thrive rather than just survive…you need others close by. You, as well as your partner, grow and flower most fully in the warmth of one another's presence. By design, not just by choice, human beings need others.

This is true from cradle to grave: the biological bond between mothers and their babies is unmistakable, primitive, and compelling; its depths know no bounds. And this is where Bowlby began his work. He discovered that a mother's consistent, persistent, attuned presence with her baby was the atmosphere the baby needed to grow and thrive (Bowlby 1982). The importance of this bond has been affirmed by researchers over many decades. It's also clear that this relationship has positive benefits for the mother too. Reciprocity is part of sustainable connection.

And it doesn't stop with infancy. Even as the baby moves through childhood and adolescence, the importance of the bond continues. The connection with their other parent and other supportive adults matters too.

When it's done well, that attachment offers security and connection. Attachment theory contends that you need a secure base to explore from and a safe haven to return to as you navigate the wonders and challenges of being a human being. This is true not only for children, but for adults too. You're never too old to need connection.

## Attachment and You

In the aftermath of betrayal, the previous section may have been difficult to read. Take a few minutes. No need to rush.

When you're ready, look at your relationship through an attachment lens. This is important work.

Think back to the time when you met your partner, fell in love, and created a life together. Recall some of the joy, excitement, and connection that entered your life. You felt alive. This was where you wanted to be. Who you wanted to be with. Clear and compelling…this was your path. This is the adult version of the attachment Bowlby studied with moms and babies. And while you're not helpless and dependent on others to physically survive as babies are, your need for closeness, connection, and security is every bit as compelling. And when you have it, you thrive; when you lose it, you don't. In attachment theory, the experience of being without a sense of closeness, connection, and security with your partner is referred to as *primal panic*.

Your partner's infidelity has likely left you feeling alone, distressed, even adrift. Primal panic is not about weakness, codependency, or immaturity. It's a natural reaction to losing the connection, the relationship you've organized your life around.

Primal panic can take many shapes. You may experience an initial sense of disbelief, confusion, and even disorientation. It's difficult to think straight. Your body may collapse. A cluster of emotions explodes: anger, rage, fear, terror. Deep pain is accompanied by hurt, sadness, and hopelessness. You may feel the impulse to lash out and at the same time want to cling to your partner. It's traumatic! And when the pain is too great, a common thought is, *Never again! I'll never let you hurt me like this again!* The intensity of your reaction indicates that the hurt you feel is more than a surface wound, something that will naturally heal over time. It's an injury—an attachment injury. The foundation you once "knew was solid and forever" has been shattered.

If you are to move forward, you'll need to heal. Self-care and connection with trusted others, family, and friends are part of the process. If your relationship is to move forward, part of your healing must occur with your partner. This calls upon your partner to step up. You need them to be present with your emotions. To hear your pain, answer your questions, and develop a sense of compassion for you. Additionally, you need them to take full responsibility for the betrayal without shifting it onto you. They also need to actively provide evidence of transparency and create safe boundaries to quell your primal panic.

The betrayal of infidelity has destroyed the security of your bond with your partner. The *secure attachment* you felt has now become insecure. Secure attachment, simply stated, is the feeling or "knowing" that your partner is there for and with you. The sense that you can count on them in good times and in bad, perhaps especially in the bad. When you need them, they'll be there by your side. When you feel alone, they show up. You "know" you matter to them. Their words and actions confirm this belief. *Insecure attachment* then leaves you in a different place. Deep inside you "know" your partner can't be trusted. You wish you could trust them, but you can't. You can't risk really depending on them. Perhaps they'll be there for you, perhaps not. Even if they do show up, is it real? This sense that your partner isn't really there for you creates an aloneness. There's nothing you can really count on. Your future together is not a given. You no longer interact under the calming, bonding assumptions of trust and commitment.

> ### Exercise: **Assess Your Attachment**
>
> *These questions are for the HP.*
>
> Respond to these questions in your journal. Describe how you felt before the betrayal was discovered.
>
> - How connected did you feel to your partner?
> - Did you feel you really knew them?
> - Did you feel they really knew you?
> - Were you able to share your life worries and concerns with them?
> - Did they do so with you?
> - When you did share with them, were they open and interested? Or did you feel a lack of interest or presence?
>
> Agree to a time to discuss your responses with your partner. If it's too early, perhaps discuss them with a friend or confidant.

## The Pillars of a Healthy Relationship

Healthy, romantic relationships aren't really complicated. Actually, they're quite simple—but simple doesn't mean easy. To recover and rebuild a relationship in the wake of betrayal, the pillars of trust and commitment must be rebuilt. These common descriptors of healthy relationships are more than just words; they're processes that must be created and lived. Not just during the crisis, but day-to-day for the rest of your life.

### Trust: Can I Count on You?

How do you define trust? A feeling inside you? A behavior or set of behaviors you or your partner do? Something you believe in or aspire to but can't describe? A statement of intent or a vow about future behavior?

Well, John and Julie Gottman have an answer. From their years of working with couples, they assert that trust is a particular state that exists when both partners in a relationship are willing to change their own behavior for their partner's benefit. Rather than making choices based solely on their own preferences or self-interest, they also take their partner's wants, wishes, and needs into consideration. They consider how their decisions will impact their partner (Gottman 2011).

Do you see evidence of this in your relationship? Do you have the feeling, *I know you've got my back. You're there for me, here with me*? When your partner makes a decision or takes an action, do they do so with full awareness and concern for how it will affect you? Perhaps the short answer to "what is trust?" is "thinking for two."

This doesn't mean that you automatically sacrifice your wants, wishes, and needs at the altar of your partner's needs. You have your own needs too. It means that when you perceive your wants to be different, perhaps even incompatible, that you'll come together to discuss them in an open, collaborative manner. The conversation will look for a way to satisfy both partner's needs. It's a collaborative way of thinking. This then becomes a guide as you go through life.

In the wake of a betrayal, trust takes on an additional quality. To begin, your partner must *earn* your trust. It's no longer something you can simply give. They need to do the work to regain your trust. It's not an even playing field. Without trust, there is no rebuilding. No path to intimate connection.

## Exercise: Exploring "Trust" In Your Relationship

*This exercise is for the HP.*

Respond to these questions based on how you felt *before* the betrayal was discovered. Use your journal.

- How did you define or describe trust?
- List three examples of times you trusted your partner and they were there for you.

> - List three times when you trusted your partner and they let you down or they weren't there for you.
> - Was there a specific moment when trust in your partner was damaged?
> - How did you respond to that situation?
> - Were you able to really talk about it or did it remain unsettled?
> - Do you believe your partner trusted you?
>
> Agree to a time to discuss your responses with your partner. If it's too early, perhaps discuss them with a friend or confidant you value.

## Commitment: Do You and Will You Always Choose Me?

Commitment is a controversial term. How do you define it? Is it a feeling inside you? An abstract value you believe in, but can't describe? A pattern of behavior, a way of acting? Is it a promise or something more? How about a decision? The decision to invest.

The research of Caryl Rusbult brings clarity to this issue. She found that "committed partners," those who did not stray and remained loyal to their partners, displayed some specific qualities. They invested in their partner and their relationship. And over time, as they continued to invest, their bond grew stronger. Their commitment deepened (Rusbult, Agnew, and Arriaga 2011). This meant they cherished their partners and experienced gratitude for what they had in their relationship as opposed to nurturing resentment for what they didn't have and internally "trashing" their partners. This cherishing led them to care about how their partner felt, and at times, to willingly sacrifice for the relationship. Over time, they were not only content to be with their partner, they even felt fortunate to be with them. Perhaps not winning-the-lottery happy but in the same ballpark.

This quite naturally left them feeling, *There's no one I would rather be with, I'm glad I chose you, you're irreplaceable!*

Does this mean everything is perfect? Hardly. But it does mean that you're "my person." When we hit a bump, we lean in and face it with kindness and respect knowing we'll get through it together. Putting in the effort, doing the work necessary to develop and maintain these qualities within a relationship doesn't happen by chance—it's intentional. It's the result of decisions you make and the work you do. It's not just fate.

### Exercise: **Exploring "Commitment" in Your Relationship**

*This exercise is for the HP.*

Respond to these questions based on how you felt *before* the infidelity was discovered. Use your journal.

- Describe what you meant by commitment. What was it? How did you know it's there?
- List three times when you felt your partner showed real commitment to you. Be specific.
- Select the most important of these moments. How did it feel? How did you respond to that incident?
- List three times when you felt your partner wasn't committed to you. Be specific.
- Select the most important one of these moments. How did it feel? How did you respond to that incident?
- Were you able to really talk about it or did it remain unsettled?

Agree to a time to discuss your responses with your partner. If it's too early, perhaps discuss them with a friend or confidant you value.

## Betrayal or Loyalty? They Don't Coexist

Your partner's betrayal was more than an oops moment or an innocent mistake. While the act of infidelity may occur in a moment of opportunity, it's typical that the seeds have taken root and grown over time.

Betrayal emerges from the toxic combination of self-centeredness as well as a conscious or subconscious win-lose mentality. This win-lose mindset takes the form of focusing on meeting their own needs, of getting the best deal for themselves regardless of how it might impact you. It's about their gain even if it causes you pain. Does this mean it was intended to hurt you? Perhaps not. But the possibility that it might hurt you was not enough to stop it from happening.

So just where does the path to betrayal begin? Once again, let's return to the work of Caryl Rusbult. One of her central discoveries was that the root of betrayal is found in the concept of *negative comparisons*. Her research found that partners, at some level, internally compare the benefits they receive from being with their partner to the benefits they *might* receive in another, real or imagined, relationship (Rusbult 1998). These "negative comps" foster a mindset of partial rather than full investment. This leads to noticing and focusing on things you consider negative about your partner. And as you spend more time there, these negative things expand in your mind. What started as a minor annoyance becomes a personal quality you can't stand. As you nurture these negative perceptions of your partner, even more negative thoughts follow. This can create resentment. This is in dramatic opposition to the cherishing and gratitude that are characteristic of fully invested partners.

Over time, this internal landscape may shift in favor of a real or imagined other. *There must be someone out there who would be less demanding, critical or needy. Someone who doesn't want to fight all the time. Someone who would be more agreeable, appreciate my humor, and even like me.* The idea of finding a person who would "meet more of my needs" gains traction. And in this mindset, there's little concern about how it would impact you. The path to betrayal begins to materialize.

> ### Exercise: **Exploring "Betrayal"**
>
> *This exercise is for the HP.*
>
> Respond to these questions based on how you felt *before* the betrayal was discovered. Use your journal.
>
> - How did you describe or define betrayal?
> - List three times when betrayal was a worry or problem in your relationship. Be specific. Who was involved? What was the situation?
> - How did you respond to those concerns?
> - Were you able to really talk about it and come to an agreement? Or did it remain unsettled?
> - Describe other times you experienced betrayal in your life.
>
> Agree to a time to discuss your responses with your partner. If it's too early, perhaps discuss them with a friend or confidant you value.

## Loyalty

After discussing betrayal, the concept of loyalty comes into focus. Loyalty and betrayal don't coexist (Gottman and Gottman 2018). And to be clear, loyalty involves much more than just not actively betraying your partner. Loyalty adds another element in healthy, sustainable relationships. Loyalty is an active, even proactive quality. It's more than a feeling within. It's a sense of caring that moves you to action when the situation calls for it. When your partner is under duress or feeling threatened, challenged, or criticized by someone, by anyone, you step up and step in (Marano 2023). You're there for them, with them. You're willing to stand up for them, to fight for them. And you do so not because you have to, but because you're moved by their distress and you want to assist them. It contains elements of support and respect, but it's based in the desire to protect. In this regard, loyalty is also part of trust and commitment, but here, it has an active, even activist, component. It's the opposite of the destructive quality of betrayal.

Just as betrayal reflects a moral code, or lack thereof, loyalty too is based on a moral code. That code calls you to come to the aid of your distressed partner, not to leave them alone in a difficult moment. When they experience a threat, you respond because you love them. The deliberation is simple: *You need me, I respond.*

So, what does this look like in everyday living? Loyalty conveys the message "I've got your back" as well as "I choose you over all others," which are core components of trust and commitment.

When in the presence of others, that protective instinct scans for danger. Without conscious awareness, you're naturally attuned to your partner and their emotional state. When they feel threatened, you sense it and respond.

Another aspect of loyalty is obvious when you're in social situations. This might involve family, friends, neighbors, or business colleagues. How do you treat your partner in front of others? When your partner speaks, do you show respect and interest or do you seem unaware of them? Worse yet, are you dismissive of their thoughts, feelings, and opinions? Do you show the world "I have your back," "I choose you over all others," or not? Does this mean you're joined at the hip 24-7? Of course not. But it does mean you're aware of and attuned to your partner.

When in private, when no one else is looking, the same idea applies. Are you engaged, invested, and committed to your partner or not? When they reach for you, seeking a moment of connection, do you take the time to focus on and engage them, or do you relegate them to the back burner?

> ### Exercise: **Exploring Loyalty in Your Relationship**
>
> *This exercise is for the HP.*
>
> Respond to these questions based on how you felt *before* the betrayal was discovered. Use your journal.
>
> - How did you describe loyalty?
>
> - List a time when loyalty was a problem in your relationship. Who was involved? What do you wish your partner would have done?
>
> - List a time when your partner stood up for you when you were being treated poorly. Who was involved? What did your partner do?
>
> - Now think of a future situation that might arise. How would you like your partner to respond?
>
> Agree to a time to discuss your responses with your partner. If it's too early, perhaps discuss them with a friend or confidant you value.

# In Closing

Here you were able to step away from the distorting lens of infidelity and revisit the central components of a healthy, loving relationship. The kind of relationship you desire and deserve. Your emphasis on trust, commitment, and loyalty will serve as a guide as you move forward. Being clear about the destructive impact of betrayal is another valuable lens.

The next chapter addresses forgiveness. In the wake of infidelity, it's a central issue.

# Part 2

# The Decision to Forgive and Communication Skills for the Journey

This is a pivotal section. Chapter 4 offers a guide to understanding forgiveness. Both you and your partner have individual work to do and issues to address. Your work here determines if you're ready to continue the journey. If you decide to move forward, chapter 5 then presents essential communication skills you'll need stay on track as you work to rebuild your relationship.

CHAPTER 4

# The Decision to Forgive

Forgiveness is a deeply personal thing. There's no easy path to it. What you decide today may not hold tomorrow. Be kind to yourself. Be patient with yourself. Reserve the right to honor your feelings, to trust your instincts, and to change your mind even if it's over and over again. Ambivalence is just part of the process. It's completely normal for a "yes" today to be followed by a "no" tomorrow. It's to be expected.

So, why is this so difficult? Well forgiveness is just complicated. In moments like these, emotions run deep, and there's a lot on the line for you as well as for those you love. Forgiveness, and the decision to stay in this relationship or not, has huge implications for your future. There's no need to rush to a final decision on whether you forgive your partner or not. Slow down, let the dust settle, and look to the future with a calm brain and clear eyes.

## Understanding Forgiveness

Forgiveness is a complicated thing. Well, it's not just one thing, it's many things:

It's a decision as well as a process.

It happens in a moment. And it unfolds over a lifetime.

It's something given and something earned.

It's a gift to yourself and a gift to your partner.

While forgiveness is many things, there is one thing it's not: simply *forgetting* (Spring 2022). There is no reset button that wipes the slate clean, that puts you back to the time before the betrayal.

It's not something you do once and then it's done. Every time the pain of the betrayal returns, the question of forgiveness comes with it. And with it, the need to forgive your partner over and over, to forgive yourself over and over. Betrayal is now part of your experience, part of your path. It has a place in the story of your relationship.

While you can't "unring the bell," you can use it as a call to action. As an opportunity to take an honest look at your relationship.

## A Decision and a Process

Your initial decision to forgive may contain many feelings. Perhaps it contains your love for your partner, the good times you've shared, the children you've brought into the world, and the joy you share over them. These experiences can be compelling. Or your decision to forgive could come from the fear of losing your partner or the life you have created together. There's a natural fear of loss, a dread of the unknown that gives you pause. This instinctive move to retain a sense of stability and minimize further loss is more common than not. The primitive fear of being alone, the uncertainty of life without your partner, is powerful. The confidence that you can work it out, that you can overcome this crisis, may also guide your decision. There are many themes that are part of the decision to forgive.

The process between you and your partner is also part of the equation. That is, their ability to see you and how you feel and their commitment to you and to the process of repair. When your partner sees your distress, do they come to you or do they remain silent? Do they attempt to sooth you, to reassure you of their love and commitment? Or do they leave you alone in your pain? Their reaction to your emotional experience may have a powerful impact on your willingness or capacity to forgive.

## Forgiveness: A Moment and a Lifetime

In some moments, forgiveness may seem to be the obvious choice. At times you may feel there's so much worth fighting for, worth preserving, and the cost of not forgiving or ending the relationship would be so devastating that it would just make matters worse. In such moments, the choice of forgiveness carries the day.

At other times, it may be equally clear that forgiveness is the wrong choice. How can you have a happy, stable life together when you can't even trust your partner to respect the fundamental integrity of your relationship? Let alone be attentive to you and value your wants, wishes, and dreams?

And whatever your decision in a given moment, your feelings can change over time. The moments of "yes, our relationship is worth it" or "no, the hurt is just too much to bear" accumulate, and the correctness of any one decision feels different based on the path you create.

## It's Given and It's Earned

At times, forgiveness begins as an act of giving grace. Grace may be a value you live by—a moral conviction, perhaps, or a religious belief. It may be supplemented by an idea that your partner is basically a good person who made a horrible mistake or the idea that we all deserve a second chance when we do something wrong. These ideas and beliefs come from within you. They're part of how you try to live your life. This kind of grace can be a wonderful starting point, and it will take something more for it to feel right. For it to move from an ideal or belief to a felt experience.

For forgiveness to become a true, genuine, sustainable feeling, it's something that also needs to be earned by the person being forgiven. That is, it can't *just* be something you give. Your partner must express real compassion for your hurt and remorse for their actions. More than just talking the talk, they must walk the walk. And they must do so not just now, during the crisis of the discovery of infidelity, but over the course of your life together. Whenever the pain resurfaces, tomorrow or a decade from now, they need to continue to earn your forgiveness.

## A Gift to Yourself and A Gift to Your Partner

Yes, a move toward forgiveness is also a gift to yourself. Stepping away from focusing on the betrayal may offer you moments of peace. Not permitting resentment to contaminate your inner landscape will add to your well-being.

Remember that you have no obligation to forgive your partner; your willingness to try to forgive is a significant gift to them. Your openness to try to go through the process of rebuilding a strong, personal, intimate bond with your partner is an act of courage and faith. It must be recognized and appreciated.

## The Decision

At this point in your recovery, forgiveness relates to a very basic question: Are you ready to make the decision to even *try* to make your relationship whole again? To try to put the pieces back together in a way that's real and healthy? That's emotionally engaged, open, and sustainable? At its core, it's a decision to try to step out of the pain, fear, and hopelessness of the present and into the possibility of a future of hope and happiness.

It's also true that living with resentment and bitterness will destroy you and take a toll on those you love. Forgiveness is good for you as well as good for your partner. It's reassuring for your children and calming for your families. Perhaps the question before you is "What type of forgiveness is right for me?"

You have the privilege and responsibility to decide what's right for you. And with that decision, you also retain the right to change your mind. Today, you can decide to try. And over time, it may feel good enough, it may feel like the right thing, or it may feel like the damage is just too great.

Keep in mind that forgiving your partner does not mean you've decided to stay with them. You can forgive your partner for the betrayal—make the choice to let go of resentment—and still decide it's too much to live with and that the relationship is no longer right for you. You can also forgive and be unable to trust your partner. And without trust, perhaps it's not the right relationship for you.

Not forgiving is not the same thing as being unfair, petty, or vengeful. You don't owe your partner forgiveness. Only you can decide if you can forgive, and what type of forgiveness is right for you.

> ### Exercise: Am I Ready to Try?
>
> *This exercise is for the HP.*
>
> Please write your responses in your journal.
>
> - List your primary reasons for being willing to work on your relationship.
> - List and describe the top three things you need in order to feel good about trying to restore your relationship.
> - List your doubts or concerns about deciding to try to repair and reconcile.
> - What is your greatest fear or worry about this?

## Do We Have a Future?

This is a time for truth telling, *real* truth telling, to yourself. It's the time to summon your courage and look at what you know to be true about your partner and if they value you and your relationship. Your response to this exploration doesn't dictate whether you'll stay or go. That's a different question. That's of course up to you. It merely invites you to be as objective and honest as you can with yourself as you make that decision. It's a time to look at all you know about your partner. From your years together before the betrayal. And what you've learned about them through how they've responded to the betrayal.

Can you trust them enough to try again or is it just too risky? Do you believe your partner will really change? Do you believe they're capable of this level of change? Do you believe that deep inside they even want to change? And by change, I mean not just to not cheat on you again, but do they truly care about how you feel? Will they be there for you, with you, in times of need? Do they want a real relationship with you?

Perhaps the most telling information is how they've responded to the shock, confusion, and distress you've experienced in response to the affair.

Are they stepping up to the moment—taking responsibility for what they did, seeking to understand how you feel, seeking to know what can be done to repair—or are they still focused on themselves and downplaying your pain? Are they touched by your struggle or more focused on justifying themselves?

> ### Exercise: **Do You See Me?**
>
> *This exercise is for the HP.*
>
> Please respond to the following questions:
>
> - Describe a time when your partner was able to step out of their own experience and step into yours. What did they say? What did they do?
>
> - Describe a time when your partner was not able to step out of their own experience and step into yours. What did they say? What did they do?
>
> - What leads you to feel hopeful or hopeless about this?

## What Is Your Goal?

You may perceive your partner as really caring, really trying, or perhaps just going through the motions. It's one thing to forgive. You may accept the idea that the betrayal was not intended to hurt you. Perhaps you can see it as a weakness on the part of your partner, a mistake or bad judgment. It's quite another to decide to move forward together. To dedicate your future to them. There are many possible paths.

Do you see a path to becoming an intimate, connected, committed couple again?

Or perhaps you're not sure that's possible. If that's the case, what do you see as possible? What might feel right to you? For instance, you might feel that the "best interests" of your kids is your top priority. But just what that looks like is another matter. It might lead you to decide to stay together.

On the other hand, it could lead you to decide to separate or divorce and really focus on working collaboratively for the kids.

> ### Exercise: Define Your Starting Position
>
> *This exercise is for the HP.*
>
> Take some time to think through this list of options. Each position brings certain benefits, as well as carrying certain risks. What you choose today may change tomorrow, but it's important to define your starting position.
>
> Are you committed to…
>
> - Staying together and rebuilding your relationship with the intention of spending your life with your partner?
> - Staying together and working on your relationship, hoping that it will work but reserving judgment?
> - Working on your relationship, seeing what's possible, but not yet sure if it's possible to stay together?
> - Working on developing a friendship and learning to communicate better? Perhaps staying together or perhaps not?
> - Processing the betrayal with no future direction in mind?
>
> Use your own words to describe your starting position.

## Forgiving Yourself

And, as the HP, there's also a type of forgiveness you need to offer yourself. Perhaps forgiveness for not noticing, accepting too little, or tolerating too much. Maybe for being too conflict-avoidant or withdrawing from the relationship. It could be the generic forgiveness of not being perfect. But remember, even if you were perfect, that's no guarantee the betrayal wouldn't have happened. In a very real sense, the betrayal wasn't about you.

## Exercise: What Do You Regret?

*This is for the HP.*

Please respond to the following questions:

- Do you feel you betrayed yourself in some way? Describe it.
- Did you lose of part of yourself, of the person you believed you were, of the values you follow?
- What do you wish you had paid more attention to?
- What would you have done differently?

*This is for the IP.*

As the partner who engaged in the betrayal of infidelity, you too have work to do. What do you want for the future? Do you see the possibility of a close, connected life together, or does it feel too late?

## What Is Your Goal?

Your life too has been drastically altered. The disruption and chaos your infidelity created has changed your relationship and altered your future. Now, as you sort through the damage, do you even know what you want?

Since the discovery of your affair, has your perspective changed? Do you have remorse and regret, or are you more upset that you got caught? Do you want a life with your partner or are you already gone? Perhaps you're not sure. Maybe you're ambivalent.

If you do want a life together, can you see any possibility of getting through the current situation and building a relationship that would be connected and sustainable? Are you willing to put in the work? These are uncomfortable but necessary questions to face.

Not being ready to leave or divorce is not the same thing as choosing your partner again. If you're uncertain, ambivalent, or leaning away from the relationship, you owe it to your partner to be honest about how you feel.

It's time to really explore not only if you want to stay but why. Of course it's okay to stay together for the kids, for financial reasons, your religious beliefs, or what your family or society would think. The reality is that not all relationships are founded in a deep personal connection or romantic love. At the same time, some people feel that a close personal bond is essential; obligation, responsibility, or propriety alone are not enough. Whatever your position, it takes courage to have this discussion, look at the options, and make the best decision for yourself and all involved parties.

## Exercise: Define Your Starting Position

Take some time to think through this list of options. Each position offers certain benefits as well as carrying certain risks. What you choose today may change tomorrow, but it's important to define your starting position.

Are you committed to…

- Staying together and rebuilding your relationship with the intention of spending your life with your partner?

- Staying together and working on your relationship, hoping that it will work but reserving judgment?

- Working on your relationship, seeing what's possible, but not yet sure if it's possible to stay together?

- Working on developing a friendship and learning to communicate better? Perhaps staying together or perhaps not?

- Processing the betrayal with no future direction in mind?

Use your own words to describe your starting position.

## Forgiving Your Partner

While this idea may seem odd in the wake of your betrayal, there may be wounds and hurts you've accumulated in your relationship. You may feel upset and resentful toward your partner. Can you face those feelings and forgive your partner for hurts you've felt over the years? Can you forgive them for the ways they contributed to your pain? Do you carry hurts or injuries that need to be healed?

## Exercise: My Injuries

Use your journal to respond to the following questions:

- Describe a moment when you felt hurt by your partner that still bothers you. What happened?

- Did you address it with your partner? What did you feel? What did you need?

How do you wish you had handled it?

## Remorse and Self-Forgiveness

As the Involved Partner, your infidelity was a betrayal of your relationship. You broke an agreement and kept it secret. In order to help your partner recover and to build a loving, sustainable relationship, you have work to do. It begins with honestly facing yourself and owning what you did. At a very basic level, do you experience remorse, not only for hurting your partner, but also for violating your own values? Remorse carries a sense of sadness and accepting responsibility for your actions. If this is you, then self-forgiveness is an important step in recovering your sense of being an honorable person. This is a very different starting position from feeling regret about being caught. To be clear, self-forgiveness is very different from self-justification.

> ### Exercise: **Remorse and Self-Forgiveness**
>
> Respond to the following questions:
>
> - Did you violate your beliefs or values in some way? Describe it.
> - Did you lose part of yourself or betray the person you believed you were?
> - Do you feel remorse? Describe what you feel remorse about.
> - Do you believe you did anything that requires self-forgiveness?
> - What do you wish you would have done differently?

# In Closing

You've started the task of understanding and addressing forgiveness: what it is and what it isn't. You've addressed where you stand and whether you're ready to begin to move forward. If you've decided that you're interested in seeing what's possible between you and your partner, it's time for the next chapter. The next step is to help you develop the communication skills required for the journey.

CHAPTER 5

# Essential Communication Skills

In the last chapter, you explored forgiveness and your readiness to take the leap to move forward together. The decision to try to reconcile and to try to rebuild your relationship is a major step. The key questions here were:

Do you even want to work on your relationship?

Is your partner someone you want a future with?

Even if the answer was a clear "yes," another question surfaced:

Are you ready to begin?

While knowing that your decision is to reconnect and rebuild offers direction, knowing how to go about it is another matter. The journey, founded in positive intent and fueled by hope, can be complicated. At times the path feels daunting.

In this chapter, you'll work on the communication skills required for the journey.

## Your Emotional Style: Expressive or Dismissive

Let's begin by looking at your communication styles. Over the course of your time on this planet, you and your partner have developed ways of thinking about and handling emotions as they occur inside you. You may tend to express your emotions, or you may keep them private. You lean toward either expressing what you're feeling or keeping those feelings to yourself. You might be considered "emotionally expressive" or "emotionally dismissive" (Gottman and Gottman 2024).

The term "meta-emotions" references how you feel about feelings (Gottman, Katz, and Hooven 1997). It's related to how you feel about experiencing and expressing emotions. This is not something you're born with. It's the result of your lived experience and interactions with the important people in your life. You might think of it as programming. Your experience as a child, adolescent, and young adult, through your current stage in life, have informed you about the benefits and perils of the emotional world. Did life teach you that emotions were good or bad, safe or dangerous, or should be expressed or suppressed?

Or perhaps you've internalized one approach to positive emotions—"by all means, let's talk about the good experiences of your day"—but another to negative emotions—"I just don't have the energy to hear one more word about your problems or unhappiness."

Even more specifically, within the realm of what we call negative emotions, you might have one approach to anger and another to sadness or fear. For example, anger feels valid and respectable, but sadness and fear are indicators of weakness.

This single issue, how you build emotional expression into or out of your interactions, has a powerful impact on your level of relationship satisfaction. If you're an emotion-expressing person, conversations void of emotional content may feel impersonal or superficial. They may leave you feeling more like a roommate than a soulmate. On the other hand, if you're in the emotion-dismissing camp, interactions centering around emotions, especially negative emotions, may lead you to feel that your partner is trying to start a fight. This is particularly true if those negative emotions are about you.

Here's a final point to consider. It's not quite as simple as saying that an emotionally expressive style is better than an emotionally dismissive style. The key issue regarding emotional styles and meta-emotions is whether you and your partner are in sync. Mismatches can be the source of great frustration and disappointment. Even well-intended conversations can go poorly because of this.

# Preparing for Conversation

*Avoid avoidance.* Talking about difficult topics is a crucial part of the recovery process. Without open, heartfelt conversations, the pain and confusion of the betrayal becomes entombed within your psyche. It creates a wall between you and your partner. Avoidance is not a path. It creates a chasm. Facing the issues that have come between you is the path to connection.

*Frame of mind.* When talking about tough topics, focus on what you're hoping to accomplish. Be mindful of what you want your partner to hear, not just what you need to say. When listening, focus on their actual words; you may be hearing something different. When discussing emotional topics, these can be elusive skills.

*Rebuttal brain to receptive brain.* When you're stressed, it's common to hear through your rebuttal brain. As you take in your partner's words, your brain looks to critique or challenge their points. The shift to your *receptive brain* invites you to actively work to hear what they're trying to say. This is essential for productive conversations on difficult topics.

*Embrace full brain communication.* Emotional intelligence is the capacity to receive and process your partner's words and feelings in your head *and* in your heart. This requires a different kind of listening. It's not about tolerating or enduring your partner's words. It's not waiting until you can get your words in. It's about truly being there with and for your partner. Not an easy task under the best of conditions. It's especially challenging now.

# During Conversations

Productive interactions on difficult issues require two skill sets. The first centers around remaining psychologically and physiologically balanced during conversations, even during difficult moments. It's called self-regulation. The second skill set focuses on *how* you talk with your partner. The words you use and the tone you choose make a difference.

## Self-Regulation

Healthy conversations require two people who are emotionally present and physiologically balanced. Once either of you becomes physiologically triggered, real conversation is over. Yes, you can continue to say words, but no real communication takes place. Negative feelings escalate, words get heated, ears close, and a fight follows.

When physiologically triggered, your nervous system activates. It's called *fight or flight*, which is an instinctual reaction to perceived threat. Once the stress hormones cortisol and adrenaline have been released, you're no longer a relationship creature. You're now in survival mode. You're temporarily limited to acting in your own self-interest. One of the first things to go is your ability to see things through your partner's eyes: to hear their experience with a sense of compassion. You can't process information clearly.

This isn't evidence of being selfish or immature. It's simply your nervous system reacting to threat. It won't last forever, but you can't just wish it away. It takes time for your circulatory system to cleanse itself of the stress hormones. So, the path of wisdom? Keep an eye on yourself and how you feel. When you notice you're having trouble hearing your partner clearly, or even listening to them at all, take a break.

Once your nervous system settles, you'll be ready to resume the conversation.

## Taking a Break

In fight or flight it's difficult to think clearly, and at times, impossible. The thinking part of your brain, the prefrontal cortex, is temporarily offline. Your limbic system, the emotional center of your brain, is in charge. It's really helpful in the face of danger, like saber-toothed tiger danger, but not so much when the "danger" is an upset partner.

You need a simple way of noticing your dysregulated state, calling for a time-out, and returning to the conversation when physiologically calm. Let's call it a Brake-Break-Return ritual.

Start by paying attention to your body. How does your body respond when you get triggered? Do you notice a tightening in your chest, your shoulders? Does your heart begin to race? Does your stomach feel queasy? Perhaps you have a headache or a dry mouth? These can be signs your nervous system is activated. Having a hard time thinking clearly or finding the right words is an important social indicator. Are you yelling and unable to stop? Are you talking over your partner? Do you even care what they're saying? These can be signs of dysregulation. It's time to hit the brakes. They're also clear indicators it's time for a break.

Focus on noticing these things in yourself. Noticing them in your partner and telling them to "calm down" is rarely well received.

Next, let your partner know you're in fight or flight. This is the cue that a break is necessary. Your nervous system needs time to reset. This is more than just lowering your heart rate. You may be able to do that in a few minutes. A real physiological reset takes time, perhaps twenty minutes of uncontaminated or undistracted time. If you continue thinking about the fight, or planning your next point in the argument, the reset clock hasn't even started. Find something that's relaxing to you. Some people walk, others meditate, do yoga, read, watch a screen, or take a nap.

After hitting the brakes, taking a break, and returning to a regulated state, you're ready to continue. Now you can listen to and be receptive to your partner's points. This doesn't mean you'll agree with them, but you'll be able to hear them. A good rule of thumb is to return to the conversation somewhere between twenty minutes and twenty-four hours after taking the break (Gottman and Gottman 2024). Here's an essential but often overlooked point: before you begin the break, set a specific time you'll check in with each other. It's best if the person asking for the break initiates the "return" time. For example, "I'll text you in thirty minutes" or "It's almost midnight, let's sleep on it and talk in the morning over coffee" reduces the likelihood that your partner will feel abandoned, which then has its own retriggering effect. Sticking to this agreement, doing what you said you would do, is also essential. This ritual is not about avoiding the topic or ending the interaction. It's about completing it with both of you in a receptive brain mode.

# What Damages Communication

It's important to develop the ability to communicate openly, to say what's on your mind, in your heart, and to have your words heard and received in the spirit intended. When discussing emotional topics, miscommunication often disrupts the flow. Negative emotions find their way into your voice, your words, and your partner's ears. You become critical, they become defensive. Yet it's important to talk. Reverting to conflict avoidance will undermine your efforts to heal the hurt and rebuild your relationship. It's easy to say, "Don't be critical or defensive," but it's difficult to know how to do it.

Relationship research from the Gottman Institute addresses this issue. The most pernicious pattern of destructive relationship communication is called the Four Horsemen of the Apocalypse (Gottman and Silver 2015). Let's refer to it as the *Four Horsemen:* These are criticism, contempt, defensiveness, and stonewalling. When they enter a conversation, that interaction and the relationship itself are heading in a negative direction.

- *Criticism* involves expressing a position or a thought with an attitude of blame toward your partner—a finger pointing of sorts. It can feel like a character assault. The partner receiving the criticism feels they're viewed as the one at fault, or even more globally, that *they're* the problem in the relationship. This activates defensiveness.

- *Contempt* is similar to criticism but with an added toxic quality. Now, you feel you're being talked down to. That your partner has assumed a position of superiority. They view themselves as smarter, more reasonable, logical, or mature than you. Maybe even a better person. You might feel belittled or demeaned. This is the most corrosive of these destructive communication styles because it says, "You're not my equal." Contempt has a chilling effect on connection, a toxic impact on intimacy.

- *Defensiveness* is a natural response to criticism or contempt. It's an instinctive reaction to words that feel unfair, unjustified, or unwarranted. It can take the form of a protest or represent an attempt to stand up for yourself. It's a way of defending yourself from being poorly treated.

- *Stonewalling* is a form of defensiveness that includes social withdrawal from a hurtful interaction. You might break eye contact or look away from your partner. You try to shut out hurtful words. There's a sense of hopelessness or feeling powerless to change the flow of the interaction. It can also be an attempt to calm yourself so you don't explode. In some cases, it includes the fight or flight reaction. While it's sometimes an understandable response, it's not productive. Stonewalling cuts off communication. It eliminates the possibility of connection. Repair isn't possible.

You may have noticed that anger is not included. Anger can be expressed in a direct way that is not blaming or demeaning. "I'm really mad! I'm furious about how this affair has uprooted our life" is not criticism or contempt. It's the genuine expression of anger. Following betrayal, anger is a legitimate emotion that needs to be expressed, heard, and healed if the relationship is to be repaired.

As destructive as these communication patterns are, there is hope. There are antidotes to help you engage in healthy conversations about difficult topics.

## Keeping the Four Horsemen at Bay

When you have something important to say, say it, but in a way it will be heard. *How* you speak to one another matters. The antidote to criticism and contempt emphasizes using a *soft start-up*, which means sharing how *you* feel, about what, and what *you* need rather than emphasizing something negative about your partner (Gottman and Gottman 2024). Before you blurt a criticism or revert to contempt, slow down. Take a moment to craft the message you want them to hear. The steps are simple, but not always easy:

1. Start by *sharing how you feel.* "I feel sad, terrified, overwhelmed, angry," not by saying something about your partner such as "You're selfish, mean, uncaring," or "You're a jerk." Yes, you need to get your feelings out, and they need to be received, but describe how *you* feel instead of making a comment about your partner.

2. Then *describe the context* of your feelings. What led you to feel that way? Something like "I feel sad when I share my feelings and there's no response. I feel all alone" or "I feel mad, really mad when I see how this whole thing is hurting our kids." Your feelings now "make sense."

3. The last step is to *express your need.* A need is not a demand. It's a statement of what it will take for you to feel differently. Search for words to describe what you *do* need as opposed to what you *don't* want. It's called a *positive need.* It gives your partner a map of how they can please you. Statements like "I need you to be a better partner," "I need you to stop being a jerk," and "I need you to stop hurting me" convey strong messages, but they don't offer a clue of what you do want. Sharing words like "I need, now more than ever, to feel your caring, concern, and love for me. I need some private time with you every evening after the kids are in bed. I need to hear words about what you value about me," or "Now, as I'm struggling to see a path forward, I need to feel you care about my pain and are interested in how I feel. It would help if we could end every day with some sharing about the day." Now your partner has a map of what to do.

*Framing* is an additional skill that permits your words to be received as intended. It's prefacing what you have to say with a statement of positive intent. Framing statements like "I want to talk about this, not to start a fight, but to get past this block between us," or "I know this is difficult to talk about, but it's creating resentment in me and I need to get it out to feel closer to you," let your partner know that you value them as you enter the conversation. It brings positivity to the atmosphere. The final step is to convey respect by asking, "Is this a good time to talk? If not, we can schedule another time."

## Staying Present to Self and Other

Now, let's focus on how you respond to your partner's words. The antidotes to defensiveness and stonewalling involve remaining internally balanced and open. As your partner speaks, you may find your rebuttal brain activating. Your instinct is to shift away from what you're hearing. You might be tempted to grab the microphone and correct them. You might feel compelled to explain or justify yourself, or perhaps you simply withdraw or shut down. Sure, these are common instincts, but unfortunately, they block communication.

When defensiveness builds within, slow down and refocus on what your partner is saying. As you hear their words, look for any part of what they're saying that kind of makes sense to you. Focus on what you can agree with, even if it's just a part of what you're hearing, rather than indulging the tendency to take issue with what you disagree with. It's a matter of focus. Try to identify some common ground between the two of you. Even a small area of common ground might be enough to keep the conversation going in a productive vein.

Letting your partner know you can understand their point and see how they feel is a step out of your world and into theirs. It doesn't mean you agree with everything they're saying. It just means that now, in real time, you've shifted your attention to their experience rather than your own. From here, you might even be able to accept some responsibility for any words, actions, or inactions that are part of your partner's experience. It's not about blaming yourself. It's about validating your partner's experience.

And, of course, you may have your own feelings about the issue your partner is addressing. Your view may also need expression, but you both can't use the microphone at the same time.

When stonewalling takes over, the antidote once again involves slowing down. When you notice the feeling of distress or the desire to flee, breathe.

The task is to learn to calm yourself so you can remain present and engaged in the interaction. You might say to yourself, *Wait a minute. I'm feeling the need to run, but I have other options. I don't really agree with what I'm hearing, but my partner has the right to feel what they're feeling. I don't have to take it personally. I can stay here. I don't need to shut down.* Just a bit of physiological soothing may do the trick. *Okay, just breathe. Take in a nice, slow, deep breath. Hold it a bit, then let it out slowly, evenly. Now do it again.* And as you become skilled at this simple procedure, you can regain your inner calm and balance without shutting down.

## Accepting Influence

*Accepting influence* is the capacity to remain open and interested in your partner's experience even in moments of distress (Gottman and Gottman 2024). It's not about agreeing with their experience, it's about taking their experience in. When they take the risk of sharing heartfelt wants, wishes, or fears, you stay with them. It's not enough to just sit there and let them talk. Accepting influence is an active presence that conveys the message "What you're saying is important to me. What you're feeling is valid. I'm trying to put myself in your shoes and really take it in, to take you in." Your interest and receptivity leave them feeling heard and seen.

It's about honor and respect, not agreement. It implies a willingness to share power. You want a solution that honors and respects both of your needs.

The ability to accept influence is especially important when your partner is expressing negative feelings about you, to you. This is challenging; it requires a deep sense of compassion for your partner.

It may help to realize that beneath their negative emotions, there's often an unmet want, wish, or longing for you that they're not able to express.

Here's a communication axiom to keep in mind: "In order to be influential, you must first be influenceable." While it sounds paradoxical, the basic idea is that we're more able to listen to our partners when we feel they listen to us. When we experience them as a "wall," we stop approaching them and find a way "around them."

## Repair When You Err

Repair may be the most crucial tool in your communication arsenal (Gottman and Gottman 2024). In the everyday flow of interacting with your partner, especially regarding emotionally loaded topics, communication sometimes fails. The message sent is not the message received. Even when sent with positive intent, it may land poorly. It's perceived as being insincere or carrying an edge. The attempt to share intimate thoughts or heartfelt feelings misses the mark. In moments like these, repair is pivotal. No matter how skilled you become at soft start-ups or staying present with your partner, you will sometimes miss the mark.

When you're driving on the highway and you drift into a rumble strip, those bumps on the edge of the road that make your tires squeal, you have a decision to make. Either course correct and get back in lane or plunge into the ditch. The choice is yours. Into the ditch or back in your lane? Your next move determines where you'll end up. You're at the wheel.

Repair is like this. When you send a message and realize it wasn't well received, how do you respond? Into the ditch or back in your lane?

Effective repair is an essential skill. In some couples, a simple "I'm sorry. I shouldn't have spoken to you like that. Let me try it again" works beautifully. In others, the empathic statement "When I really think about it…you're right and I can see how you feel" does the trick. Statements like "That's a good point," "I never thought of it that way," "I might be wrong here," or "No matter what I said, I now realize I'm a big part of the problem, it's not all on you" help partners get back in lane.

When it comes to repair, acting sooner than later makes a world of difference (Gottman, Driver, and Tabares 2015). Owning the "error" of your communication *before* you dig the hole too deep matters. Speaking from the heart, addressing and expressing emotions rather than just intellect, is also important. "Okay, okay, let me jump in here. When you were telling me your view and how you felt, I got upset, turned it to anger, and jumped on you. That's on me! You didn't deserve that! In fact, you were actually making a good point. I haven't been very attentive to you lately. I've been in my own world. I was just having a hard time admitting it. *I was wrong.* I think I can listen better now. Can you forgive me?"

Here's a simple tip that means a lot but is difficult to master. Practice saying "I was wrong" with humility and sincerity.

## In Closing

As we leave this chapter, you've gotten an appreciation for some skills required for healthy communication. When you're discussing a topic as emotionally powerful as betrayal, these details matter. Keep them in mind as you work through the following chapters.

# Part 3

# Healing the Hurt and Building the Bond

Take a moment to reflect on all you've accomplished. You've done the challenging work of preparing for the journey. You're now ready to step on the field and begin the process of working through the rubble, establishing a foundation and building a relationship that is both rewarding and sustainable.

With that preparation completed, you'll now shift to directly working together on your relationship. You'll move through the Atone-Attune-Attach model together (Gottman and Silver 2012). These chapters include interactive exercises for both of you. You'll also develop the skills to help you navigate the journey.

As you do this work, remember that there's a fluidity among these three stages of healing. They're not linear. For example, even after you've worked through *atonement,* issues of transparency and verification may surface again. Before beginning the work with one another, it may be wise to read the complete section. It will offer a better perspective of the process.

CHAPTER 6

# Healing Begins with Atonement

The path to healing begins as you and your partner come together and face what has happened. While you might be tempted to try to simply move forward, to hit the reset button, without doing this work, there's risk involved with that strategy. Talking through the betrayal and coming to a clear, complete understanding of what happened and what needs to be corrected is important.

Broken trust can be likened to a shattered bone. It won't heal well unless it's treated properly. Here we'll describe the process that will treat your brokenness and set the foundation for restoring trust and building a healthy relationship. A foundation that not only creates connection, but helps you develop a sustainable, intimate bond as you walk the path together.

The atonement phase begins the healing process. It sets the groundwork for the relationship rebuilding to follow (Gottman and Silver 2012). While it starts with a focused conversation, it doesn't happen in a flash. It takes place over time, through a series of conversations. As the initial interaction answers some questions, it raises others. Uncovering and putting together the shattered pieces of your life is a complicated process, not the task of a single conversation. While it's impossible to predict how long this phase will take, it's clear that your partner's emotional presence and caring responses are essential. Their compassion and remorse fuel the journey.

## Atonement

Your trust in your partner has taken a hit. You can no longer just believe what they say. You're not confident they're doing what they say they're doing. Your emotions are activated, you're on edge and the passage of time doesn't seem to help. Sleep doesn't come easily. Superficial conversation doesn't reflect what's going on in your mind. *How could you do this to me? What were you thinking? Do I matter to you? Do we have a future together? Does my pain touch you at all?* Thoughts like these make up the symphony playing in your head. It can be deafening.

How do you silence the questions? Find moments of peace? It's not something you can do for yourself. The truth is that you need to talk! Not just chat but really talk. You need to talk and be heard. Not just listened to but truly heard! And not by just anyone, but by your partner. It's an obvious truth but sometimes a difficult one to accept; after all, they're the one who caused your pain. They're the one who betrayed you. Yet in the wake of a betrayal, when you seek to engage in a process of repair, they're the one you need. Now more than ever.

As you absorb these words, does any of it ring true? Yes, of course, you muddle through the day. You manage what must be done. You attend to your career, the kids, and everything else. You're competent and capable, but you're also struggling. You need to talk! More than anything you need to sit down with your partner and process what happened. To ask the questions that continue to haunt you that still somehow don't make sense. Yes, you've likely exchanged words about these matters, at times with tears, at others with anger, but it's likely that the responses you've received don't relieve the pain or lessen the confusion.

It's time to try again, but this time with a clear understanding of what needs to happen and how to go about it.

## The Atonement Process

Atonement is the process of dealing with the rawness of the discovery, the shattering of your foundation, and the turmoil, uncertainty, and ambivalence of the moment. Your world has been shaken. What you once knew to be true is an elusive memory. This is traumatic. And to begin the journey, you need to start a conversation about the devastating emotional impact of what's happened to you; you need to dig through the rubble and begin to piece it together. You need to be able to make sense of this life-altering experience.

*This is for the IP.*

### Remorse

The fuel that will drive this early phase of the journey comes from you, the Involved Partner (IP).

Have you arrived at the place of real remorse? Not just "sorry you caught me" or "too bad you're suffering," but the personal remorse that comes only from owning your actions and taking responsibility for the tidal waves that followed.

This may seem self-evident, that when we do something we're not proud of, or that we know is wrong, we're remorseful, but it's not a given. While the words of remorse can sometimes flow easily, true remorse is more than words. It's a shift from the thinking and justification that permitted the betrayal, to understanding and feeling the horror of what you've done, as well as the pain and trauma you inflicted on your partner, and perhaps in the disappointment you have in yourself. Without this internal shift, the surface remorse one might feel immediately after the discovery of infidelity fades.

You strayed from the relationship foundation of being open and honest with your partner. This is on you. This, in and of itself doesn't make you a bad person, but what you do with it matters. It's now on you to make it right—or at least to try. I mean really try, not mutter something about "sorry," turn away, and say, "Let's move forward."

Remorse is a fundamental shift of perspective. Not a few words of apology.

### Responsibility

Saying you accept responsibility is one thing. Living responsibility is quite another. Your remorse is the ingredient your partner needs to feel a bit of hope. Your remorse sends the message that, now in the light of day, with a clear head, you see the error of your ways. You feel the pain it created. True remorse is at the center of owning what you did, of accepting responsibility. And accepting responsibility is not just a timely phrase, it's a pattern of clear, consistent, committed behavior. It's being able to be present with your partner in their distress. Not just today and tomorrow but over the course of time.

Together, remorse and responsibility must become guiding principles to helping your partner and relationship heal from the trauma of what you've done. You don't "do" them, you *live* them. They become part of who you are and in a way that's dedicated to your partner rather than demeaning yourself.

This level of responsibility takes real courage and strength of conviction. It requires overcoming the all too human tendency to focus on your justification for the betrayal. Do you have a story to tell? A case to plead? Wants, wishes, and needs to discuss? Of course! But this is not the time. That will come later. Now is the time to stay in the reality of the trauma your partner is experiencing. To be with them. Not to leave them alone.

### *Compassion*

Remorse and responsibility permit you to be with your partner in their pain. And, as you allow their emotions and their struggle to impact you, to enter you, compassion begins to grow. Your compassion begins to stop the bleeding and heal the wound the infidelity created. Over time, it's the balm that soothes the sting. True compassion is more than something you feel inside. It's something that seeks expression: in your words and actions, in your very demeanor, you convey a sense of presence. Your partner begins to feel it, perhaps faintly at first and with considerable doubt. But, as you remain steadfast, they will feel it more strongly, more deeply. This is your challenge—your opportunity.

# The Conversation

Now it's time to have the first conversation. While conversations are exchanges between two people, this one has some specific conditions.

For the Involved Partner (IP): It's up to you to set the tone. Regardless of what you've already covered together or how many times you've tried to talk about the affair, this is another starting point. And to the extent you do this well, it will begin to have a positive impact on the tone and temperature of future interactions with your partner. But before beginning, you need to take the time to prepare yourself.

And to the Hurt Partner (HP): You too have a role to play. You need to ask the questions that are haunting you, causing you distress, that are hard to get out of your head. You have a right to know, and you deserve the answers. And to make this exchange productive, rather than just another frustrating blowout, you too have some preparation to do.

---

### *For the Involved Partner.*

As the IP, preparing yourself for atonement conversations begins with the recognition that your partner is in crisis. They're not just upset but in an actual crisis state, a state of trauma. Intense emotions are to be expected and respected. It's your responsibility, or perhaps you can see it as an opportunity, to truly be there for your partner. This is not about keeping your mouth shut and tolerating their emotions. It's about being interested, engaged, and letting them know you hear them and care about them.

So here are a few tips:

- Shift your focus away from yourself. The next few minutes are not about you!

- Turn off your "rebuttal brain." Don't evaluate what they say, just take it in.

- Make it your agenda to hear their words and try to understand their experience.

As you listen to their pain and their feelings, allow yourself to see how their reactions are understandable. When you see things differently or have a different memory of a given moment, stay with their feelings. Don't revert to yours. You don't have to agree with them to have compassion for them.

> This kind of emotional presence requires a clear mind and a calm nervous system. Even if this isn't your typical way of communicating, you're capable of it. It's your concern for and caring about your partner that makes this possible. It just takes a little selflessness and a bit of practice. In difficult moments, remember: just breathe. If you're invested in the process of repairing your relationship, you'll make it through these conversations.

For you, as the HP, your preparation also begins with the recognition of crisis, but the task before you is different. Take a moment and breathe a bit. Clear your mind and calm your nervous system.

In the exercise that follows, you'll be guided to come up with questions you wish to ask your partner. The questions that only your partner can answer. Take this opportunity to be as clear as you can about what you need to know. Don't worry about getting every question on paper. No matter where you start, additional questions will come to you when you talk with your partner. Here, you're preparing for an emotional discussion. Having some of your questions on paper will help. They'll serve as a guide, rather than a restriction.

Now, the difficult part. Take whatever time you need to draft the questions in a way that gets to the key points but also in a way your partner might be able to hear them. Rather than "What were you thinking, what's wrong with you?" or "What the hell is wrong with you? You selfish jerk!" look for the words that will make it more likely that you'll get the information you need. Bottom line, it's not really your responsibility to baby your partner. Regardless of how you say it, it's still their job to be truthful. I'm simply saying the words you choose will have some impact on how the conversation goes.

Given this, don't shy away from any real questions on your mind. If this relationship is to have a future, it will be fed by real talk. Addressing rather than avoiding issues is the first step.

> ## Exercise: **Prepare Your Questions**
>
> *This exercise is for the HP.*
>
> Find a quiet place to prepare ten questions that are haunting you.
>
> You might explore the facts of how the affair happened. The "when, where, how, who," kind of questions. Don't dig too deeply into the "why" at this point. That will come later. In a similar way, defer any inquiries about sexual behaviors or details about emotional intimacies. Remember, the goal is to begin a series of real conversations that will move your relationship forward, not to simply reopen the wounds.
>
> You might ask about things that just don't make sense to you. Things you simply don't believe. Knowing the truth might restore your confidence in your intuitions and observations. It's particularly difficult to move forward if you experienced gaslighting: that is, the disorienting communication strategy that tries to convince you that your perceptions, beliefs, and suspicions about your partner were ridiculous, paranoid, or even delusional when they were actually accurate. It's particularly painful to realize that the person who claimed to love you was willing to throw you under the bus to protect themselves. While these experiences can be difficult to overcome, they're essential to face if you're to get to a place of connection and intimacy.

### *Conducting the Conversation*

It's important to remember that these conversations are made of more than words. They're also made of emotional presence by the IP and self-awareness by the HP.

As the HP, remembering your preparation, it's time to approach the crisis that consumes you. The goal is to have a conversation with your partner that addresses your questions without leading to retraumatization.

# Healing Begins with Atonement

Remember you may be in a fragile state. Trauma symptoms may color your daily existence. You may be sleep deprived, hypervigilant, struggling with intrusive thoughts, or experiencing flashbacks. In your situation, this is to be expected. The betrayal cracked your foundation. Your sense of reality has been shaken.

In these tenuous moments, what you need above all else is something to hang on to. Your partner's truthful response to your difficult questions is a beginning. Once again, be kind to yourself. In the moment, only ask what you're ready to address, what you're ready to hear. There's no rush to face it all at once. There will be additional conversations.

This is asking a lot, but remember to approach your partner in a way that increases the likelihood of getting real answers to your questions. Use some of the language you crafted in preparation for this conversation. Also recall that being emotional, even expressing the depths of your anger, hurt, and fear, is not unhealthy. It's not being immature or unfair. It's more a matter of "how" you do it.

Recall what you learned about the Four Horsemen in the last chapter. You can share deep hurt, anger, sadness, fear, and disappointment without criticism, blame, or contempt. The "I feel, I need" protocol can help. And if or when one of the Four Horsemen surfaces, a simple repair can help you get back on track.

It's also important to remain mindful of your state of physiological arousal. If you become triggered, with your heart rate exceeding 100, just sit back, slow down, and take a breath. The work you did on flooding will come in handy in those moments. It may be wise to take a break. When you enter fight or flight, your nervous system acts to protect you from threat or perceived danger. With stress hormones at the wheel, you act to survive. You defend yourself. In this state you're more likely to just make things worse. A break of twenty minutes or more will be good for you as well as for your relationship.

Now, find those questions. Use them as a guide. They're not meant to limit you in any way. Just to give you a bit of grounding if things begin to feel overwhelming.

### *For the Involved Partner.*

These same cautions about the Four Horsemen and flooding also apply to you. In trying to have a real conversation about this difficult topic, you too might get triggered. This is especially true if one of your strategies was simply to avoid conflict, minimize self-disclosure, and deny, deny, deny. This is where addressing, rather than avoiding difficult moments, might lead you to feel cornered. You might feel overwhelmed. Here, your work on remorse, responsibility, and compassion are called on. Can your caring about and commitment to your partner permit you to be there for them?

### *Transparency*

Your challenge—and opportunity—is to be honest, truthful and transparent. You may be asked to address, to admit, to reveal some things that don't reflect well on you. Things that call your judgment or even your character into question. Facing what you learned to avoid will not come easily. It will not happen spontaneously. It requires change on your part: it's a 180 degree shift from the betrayal mindset of avoidance. But if you're able to gather yourself, remain in compassion, and keep an eye to the future, the courage to be truthful will find you.

Transparency goes beyond simply telling of the truth. It also moves into the territory of giving your partner what they need to begin to feel secure.

Your partner has likely been stuck in the role of continually looking for deception and inconsistencies. This is exhausting. So, it's not enough for you to simply offer a minimal response to the questions they ask. Partial truths aren't truths at all. To free your partner from the yoke of being vigilant and scanning for lies, of being an investigator, you're asked to become the guardian of truth and disclosure. You're called to give them the full story about the topics they mention. Better yet, to give them the full story about issues or situations they failed to mention. You need to make investigating unnecessary. Preemptive disclosures are the key. Don't put your partner in the position to be shocked yet again by something you didn't tell them.

Throughout it all, keep in mind: the purpose of these difficult conversations is not to judge, condemn, or villainize you. The real intent is to create a path back to your partner. A return to your true self. And a return to your relationship.

### *Verification*

In the aftermath of betrayal, you need to reestablish your credibility, your integrity. Your future relationship will be built on a foundation of new information, new experience. Now, you not only need to say the truth; you also need to verify it. Verification is the process of offering your partner the information they need to feel confident they know the truth.

This isn't about your partner calling you a liar or being insecure, it's about their nervous system doing what it was created to do: to protect them! Their nervous system needs proof that they can count on you. It's an evolutionary, survival kind of thing. Whether they ask for it or not, they need it to be able to trust you again. This is an opportunity for you to act in the best interests of your relationship, by offering them, of your own volition, what they need in order to feel safe in relationship with you.

At its core, verification is simply asking that you confirm that something is true, with data beyond your words. You've already demonstrated that there are veracity gaps there. Simply saying, "The affair is over," or that when you came home late it was because you "had to work late" isn't enough! You now need to prove it. Even if your partner wants to believe you, their self-protective, survival sensor will not be soothed by mere words. Especially if they've heard similar stories before. Now you need to offer them more. They need proof that the words are true. Of course, it's impossible to prove a negative—something you didn't do. But the more transparent you can be, and the more proof you can offer in support of what you *did* do, the more assured your partner will feel that they can trust you.

> After betrayal, verification may take the form of access to your devices. Seeing your viewing history, knowing your passwords. In life as it was before the betrayal, this might be considered a boundary violation, an invasion of privacy. Now in this post-betrayal world, it's simply the cost of rebuilding trust. Will this go on forever? Probably not. It's an uncomfortable way to live. But for now, embrace it.

## Back to the Conversation: Begin with an Apology!

A genuine apology begins with an "I'm sorry," but doesn't end there. A meaningful apology starts with admitting that *you were wrong*. It's surprising how many partners, even betraying partners, have never uttered the words "I was wrong" with any conviction. Have you said them…maybe. But without any emotion. Without specifically describing and admitting how you were wrong. Without the emotional energy that comes from deep within. Saying "I was wrong" is not simply a hoop to jump through or a box to check, it's a genuine admission based on humility and self-reflection. Your partner not only needs to hear the words but to feel your sincerity. And you need to feel that sincerity within yourself.

The next piece is to go beyond words and enter the realm of action. Actions add credence to the intent that's embodied in words. In the case of recovery from infidelity, actions are about making amends. And amends aren't about just any action. Amends are about doing the specific actions your partner needs to begin to feel more secure. The task for you is to "put your money where your mouth is." To do the things your partner needs to feel your words are genuine.

Saying "I'm sorry…I was wrong…I want to make amends" begins the process of repair. But as your conversations and the work of healing continue, it's essential you keep in mind that an apology is not just the words of a moment. It's the behavior of a lifetime.

As you begin the conversation, take a moment to reflect on your partner's apology. Does it ring true? Can you begin to believe it, at least parts of it? You might want to believe it, but you still have doubts. The depth, sincerity, and consistency of your partner's apology is telling. It's an indicator of what's possible between you.

Share how you feel. Begin with your questions. There's no way to ease into it. Today's conversation may answer some questions, fill in some gaps. It will also likely give rise to more questions. The flow of the conversation, the topics to be covered can't be fully scripted. They will be unique to you. Some will emerge from the flow. The important thing is that you traverse the course together. Moving beyond avoidance is essential.

What do you need to know? Ask about the facts of the affair—the who, when, how, and where are valid questions. How did you meet? Who is this person? How did it happen? When and where did you meet? How widely is it known? Who did you tell? Who knows about it?

Probe the things that just don't make sense to you. Perhaps things you don't believe. Stories you've been told that just don't ring true. Was that weekend away really a business trip? All five days?

You need to regain trust in your eyes, ears, and instincts. If you've not only been lied to but also experienced gaslighting this is essential. If your perceptions and suspicions have been ridiculed, if you've been treated as if you were crazy, you need to be made whole again. This isn't a luxury, it's a necessity. It's your right! There's no place for gaslighting in a healthy relationship.

It's also important to explicitly explore the issue of why your partner wants to stay in this relationship. Through the betrayal, they took the risk of losing you, of ending the relationship. Now, after the discovery, what leads them to want to rebuild? Why the change of heart? The intention of these questions isn't to challenge that decision but rather to invite them to put into words why you and your relationship are meaningful to them. Why they don't want to leave. Why they don't want to lose you.

The atonement process starts here and continues over an undetermined period of time. It's less based on the calendar than it is on the heart. As conversations answer some topics, they open others. This is to be expected. It's how genuine, sustainable healing begins. As compassion and vulnerability enter the exchange, trust, hope, and even a bit of forgiveness begin to take root.

# Exercise: Making Agreements

*This exercise is for the HP.*

As the Hurt Partner, it's important to let your partner know what kind of transparency and verification you need to try to move forward. You'll then try to come to an agreement on these complex topics. These agreements are works in progress. Your needs may, and likely will, shift over time. You'll need to revisit and revise them as you go through the process. Today's conversation is a starting point.

## Transparency Agreement

Describe what you need to know to worry less and feel more comfortable. You need to be free to ask questions as they arise and state your needs as they become clear to you. Here are some common themes:

*Fact* questions: Have you had any contact with the affair partner? Will you tell me if they contact you? Where were you, what were you doing when you didn't respond to my text?

*Feeling* questions: How do you feel about me? Do you want a life with me? Are you still thinking about the affair partner?

Just a reminder for you, the IP. Be proactive! Sharing things with your partner before they ask often has a positive impact. It helps them drop the interrogation role.

## Verification Agreement

Describe what verification you need. What issues do you need confirmation of, via data, to feel secure that they're telling you the truth?

Do you need specific information, the "data," about where they were, who they spent time with, what time they left the office, what they did while your daughter was at swimming practice?

Do you need to have access to their phone, other devices or their social media accounts?

> ### Formalize Your Agreements
>
> Write your agreements in your journals. Be specific so there aren't misunderstandings. If new conditions come up, add them to your agreements.

# In Closing

In closing, as you advance through the atonement process, there's a softening—a coming together over the pain and emotional upheaval you've experienced. Your partner's emotional presence is palpable. Their compassion and remorse, their willingness to be honest and transparent even on difficult issues, begins to build a foundation. You feel you're hearing the truth. You trust your instincts, your perceptions again. You can share your thoughts and ask questions with confidence. You experience your partner as being there for you.

And then, at some point, the possibility of moving forward together doesn't seem so foolish, so risky. You feel less vulnerable. Fully trusting? Of course not. But trusting enough to see the possibility of a future together. You notice your fear and apprehension beginning to diminish. They're not gone but perhaps less pervasive, less intense. You're beginning to forgive.

You're also feeling more ready to begin to really look at your relationship. Of course, there are issues; all relationships have issues. You now have the security of knowing that despite these issues, nothing you did or didn't do, said or didn't say caused the infidelity. Your partner had other choices. With this established, you're now free to explore your relationship issues. Patterns of interacting that emerged over time. Patterns that you, as well as your partner have participated in. The dance of your daily lives.

In the next chapter, you'll move into the *attunement* phase of recovery. Here you'll build the communication skills to be friends again. You'll learn how to have more personal conversations and have a more empathic connection. You'll also work on the skills required to face rather than avoid difficult issues.

CHAPTER 7

# Attunement: From Avoiding to Addressing Issues

Your work during the atonement phase helped you weather the storm and deal with the crisis of the discovery of your partner's infidelity. While the feelings, fears, and apprehensions remain with you, they're likely not quite so intense. Perhaps they're less intrusive. And now, you've arrived at the point that you're ready to begin the rebuilding of your relationship or at least to discover what's possible. This phase of recovery is called attunement. In it, you'll develop the relationship skills required to get to know each other again and revitalize your friendship. You'll also build the relationship muscles you'll need to address issues rather than avoid them. The focus will be on the two of you working to rise from the ashes and build a new foundation. During attunement, the focus shifts to *how* you communicate and interact with each other (Gottman and Silver 2012).

In this chapter, you'll start with the skills required to address rather than avoid important issues. Remember, avoidance leaves you more distant and disconnected.

## Attunement

Attunement begins with an interest in deepening your relationship. The goal is to learn to be truly present with your partner. To deeply listen to their feelings and experience their wants and needs. When done well, both of you will feel respected, understood, and known. The skills involved are clear, specific, and direct. They're accessible, not mysterious.

There is, however, one barrier you must overcome before working on your friendship. That old nemesis of avoidance. This part of the healing journey invites, perhaps requires, you to directly address some of the conflicts and areas of contention you've learned to moved away from. Do you have to talk about every topic, every area of difference that exists between the two of you? Well, of course not. But it does mean that any topic that feels important merits consideration. Any subject that surfaces and repeatedly returns, even without invitation, calls to be opened. Conflict avoidance is at the core of some of the processes that left you feeling disconnected and lonely. It leaves issues unresolved and needs unmet.

Another more personal issue is the avoidance of *self-disclosure*. In its simplest form, self-disclosure involves sharing your feelings and needs with your partner. Letting them know who you really are and what's bubbling inside. Here too, this doesn't mandate that you blurt every feeling or give voice to every need. What it does require, however, is that you become cognizant of your internal landscape and take your happiness seriously. It's essential that you feel your feelings and needs are valid. It's crucial that those feelings and needs are acknowledged and respected. As you share them with your partner, you shift the field of play from your inner world to the relational world. It's here that your feelings can be validated and your needs met.

Here are the core exercises to use to develop healthy interactions around difficult topics. Use the skills you worked on in chapter 5 as you move into these more complex conversations.

## Gottman-Rapoport Conversation

The Gottman-Rapoport conversation is based on psychologist Anatol Rapoport's insight that postponing persuasion efforts and focusing on understanding one another rather than influencing one another is the key to engaging in a collaborative interaction (Gottman and Silver 2012). Here you'll be asked to move away from trying to convince your partner of your position and be invited to ask them to simply understand and respect your feelings and needs. In doing so, you'll move out of self-disclosure avoidance and into sharing your feelings and needs. This exercise develops the communication skills that future exercises will build on.

In this exercise, you and your partner will be asked to hold a conversation, or multiple conversations, while taking turns as the Speaker and the Listener. While it may feel a bit artificial, the Speaker-Listener protocol provides an important structure for clear communication. In areas of tension, when you both try to express your feelings and needs at the same time, neither of you will feel listened to. You're fighting for the microphone. One or both of your voices will escalate or go silent. In either case, real communication fades. This exercise is about the vulnerability of speaking from your heart and the compassion of listening with your heart. This type of emotional presence isn't required in all of your conversations. It is necessary here as you enter the territory of discussing betrayal or other emotional issues or injuries that have damaged your bond. At the end of the day, it's about both of you feeling heard, understood and respected.

Think of a topic you would like to discuss. You'll begin as the Speaker. Start with something like "I've got a topic I'd like to talk about." Then preface it with a bit of framing like "I'm not trying to start a fight but rather want to share something with you." Adding, "Is this a good time for you?" shows respect for the other person's time, mood, or energy level. If it's not a good time for them, negotiate a time that would work for both of you. Investing a bit of awareness and thought into how and when you make your request will pay dividends. If possible, choose a time when your partner seems likely to be open to your request.

As the Listener, it's important to be sure you're in the position to be truly receptive, even curious about your partner's position. This isn't a time to debate, contest, or rebut your partner's feelings or needs. It's a time for you to be emotionally calm and present. Your role here is to simply hear your partner and take in their points and the related emotions. Your task then is to reflect back what you heard and validate your partner's position. Here's a crucial point: you don't have to agree with their positions in order to validate them. You can simply see how their perspective makes sense from their life experience. It's understandable that they would have that position.

The Speaker-Listener protocol is designed to be sure both of you have the opportunity to share how you feel and what you need about any particular topic.

If it's your topic, you start as the Speaker. Take a moment, go internal, and find words for the feelings that reside within. Focus on yourself and how you feel (*I feel frustrated, scared, overwhelmed, hopeless, mad, sad,* and the like), not on what you feel about your partner (*You're cold, selfish, controlling,* and the like). Share your feelings as clearly as possible.

Then, shift your attention to what you need. Focus on your positive need. Describe what you want, not what you don't want. "I need at least a little time with you every evening," not "I need you to stop being so self-centered and get your face out of your phone." Or, "When we talk, I need to feel you care and that I've heard the truth," rather than "I want you to stop lying to me."

It can be challenging to find the right words to describe what you actually *do* want, rather than what you *don't* want. Our minds so easily go to the negative. (There are more words for negativity than positivity in every language on our planet.) Put the effort in to discern and articulate what you *do* need as clearly as you can. It can help to think of what drives or underlies a certain behavior that hurts you or that you think is a problem. For instance, your partner's "having their face in their phone" may feel, to you, like a form of stonewalling, like they're freezing you out, when what you want from them is openness, contact, trust, and intimacy. Sharing this with them, that you need "openness, contact, trust, and intimacy," gives them a picture, or a map, of what they can do. It might then lead to conversation about what that would look like.

The Gottman-Rapoport Conversation is designed to facilitate an open exchange of feelings and needs. The focus is not so much on problem-solving as it is on being heard, seen, and understood on topics of conflict or concern. As both of you feel your partner's understanding and compassion, the path to emotional intimacy begins to open.

### Exercise: The Gottman-Rapoport Conversation

*This exercise is for both of you.*

Select a topic that carries some degree of tension, one that you recognize is causing some distress, but not one that is too hot; perhaps a four on a ten-point scale. The topic should be real but not overwhelming. Once you've mastered this process, you'll use it with more emotionally loaded topics.

Decide who will be the first Speaker and the first Listener. The person with the most hurt should consider being the Speaker. It may be difficult for that person to be the Listener until they feel heard, valued, and understood.

Select a topic and write a sentence or two to present it to your partner. You might begin with something like:

"I know this has been a difficult topic for us, but I need to talk about it again because it's not going away. I had trouble sleeping again last night. Are you willing to spend a few minutes with me now?"

Or you might opt for something as direct as "I'm having a hard time and really need to talk." Remember, the goal is to have a positive interaction, not another fight.

**Speaker's Role:** Describe your feelings and needs regarding a topic of importance. It could be about the betrayal, or it might be about another issue. Be sure to describe how you feel and be specific about your positive need. ("I need to spend fifteen minutes with you when I get home from work" as opposed to saying "You need to stop being so self-absorbed that you don't even notice when I walk in the door.")

**Listener's Role:** Reflect back the essence of what you heard your partner say. Be sure to share your understanding of their feelings and the emotional importance of the issue. Then ask your partner if you heard them correctly, if you "got it right."

At this point, the Speaker can add to their comments or confirm, "Yes, you got it right." Then try to validate your partner's experience. Validation doesn't mean you agree with their perspective. It simply means that, as you listened to their words, you were able to see how their experience makes sense. You can see why they felt the way they felt. Ideally, you were also able to find some compassion for them and feel motivated to try to meet their need.

You can then genuinely say something as simple as "You know honey, I didn't quite see this so clearly before, but now that I was able to really take it in, I totally see why you feel that way. I'm so sorry I'm putting you through this. You don't deserve that."

After a positive interaction over a tense topic, you might spend a bit more time deepening your understanding. Give connecting moments space to breath and time to sink in.

Then change roles and allow the Listener to become the Speaker. You may decide to do the second part of the exercise immediately, or

> depending on the moment, you might opt to take a break before trading roles. When you begin the second part of the interaction, be sure it's not a rebuttal to the first. It's not about making a point or convincing your partner of your point of view. It's simply about going inside and sharing feelings and needs that let your partner know and understand you.
>
> Remember, this exercise can be used with a wide range of topics. The basic intent is to create moments of clear, noncontentious communication where you both feel heard and understood. Practice the Gottman-Rapoport Conversation using a real but not too emotionally loaded topic.

## Don't Permit Fights to Fester

Another central task of the attunement phase is to be able to process difficult interactions: interactions that left you feeling alone, misunderstood, and uncared for. Unprocessed fights add bricks to your backpack. They add to the weight you carry, to the burden you feel in day-to-day life. Again, this calls on you to push through the tendency to avoid and to gather the courage to have a conversation about the fight. The goal is to revisit the fight and open the feelings from it without having the fight all over again.

As both of you understand more about your partner's feelings and experience of the fight, the negative energy begins to dissipate. The narrative that emerges adds to your understanding of their experience. You begin to see them differently. For example, rather than seeing them as trying to hurt you, you realize that they were desperately trying to protect themselves. They were feeling unloved, vulnerable, and at risk, then responded in an angry, attacking manner. In real time, they felt it was all your fault. They felt they were innocent, that you were the villain. You might have had similar feelings.

When moments like these are unprocessed, they are absorbed into the core of how you feel about your partner and perhaps more importantly, how you feel they feel about you. This leaves you feeling alienated and disconnected.

The following exercise is a guide to revisiting the fight and talking through it without restarting it. Processed fights carry less negativity into the future. In the best case, well-processed fights bring you closer together.

> ## Exercise: Aftermath of a Fight or Regrettable Incident
>
> *This exercise is for both of you.*
>
> Select a fight or disagreement that went poorly, leaving you feeling mistreated, unappreciated, and unseen. An interaction that fed the idea that your partner doesn't really care about you, or perhaps even left you feeling they're selfish or mean. These are the kind of fights that need to be processed. Left unchecked, they do great damage to your relationship.
>
> Spend a few minutes discussing the fights to consider. It's important that you come to a consensus here. Deciding on the fight to process should not become another fight. This is another conversation that asks you to follow the Speaker-Listener protocol. It's just too difficult to have an unstructured conversation about an interaction that caused so much pain. Remember the goal is to process the fight, not to restart it.
>
> The requirement to effectively reopen and process a fight without re-entering it is simple. You both need to recognize that you're not working on one fight, you're addressing *two* fights. The one that is etched in your memory and resides within you and the one living inside your partner. While these fights have some similarities, they also have significant differences. Who was the protagonist? The antagonist? Who started it? Who escalated it? Who refused to let it drop? What were the critical moments? You would both respond to these questions differently. You both carry a different movie in your head about what happened. Those movies are the narratives you believe to be true. Your experiences and perceptions create powerful memories that aren't easily dismissed. If given a lie detector test, you would easily pass, as would your partner. No one can talk you out of your lived experience. To try is an exercise in futility.

What can be addressed, however, is how you look at the fight, or regrettable incident, upon review. By engaging in this exercise, you can both begin to see it through different eyes. Through more compassionate eyes. This perspective shift won't erase the fight from your memories, but it will change how you look at it and the meaning you assign to it. You may see your partner in a more compassionate light.

Before beginning this exercise, breathe for a moment. Now prepare yourself to hear about your partner's experience of the fight. Each step in this process sounds simple, and they are; they're just not easy. To the extent you can create space for their movie, you'll be able to reduce the negative residual effect of the fight.

The flow of this exercise is that you and you partner take turns responding to each question before moving to the next step. For example, both of you will complete step one by sharing the feelings you experienced in your movie before moving on to the next step.

Since this exercise is about discussing a conflict between you and your partner, it carries a certain amount of negative emotion. You might feel angry, resentful, or sad—to name a few of the many possible emotions. Before beginning, take a few deep breaths to calm your nervous system. Remind yourself of the communication skills discussed in chapter 5. Prepare yourself to listen, to really hear your partner's experience even though it differs from yours. Move out of your rebuttal brain and into your receptive brain. You don't need to agree with them, you simply need to understand and respect their feelings and experience. If you listen well enough, you might even begin to notice a bit of compassion for them welling up inside you.

## Step One: Sharing Your Feelings

Take a moment to recall the feelings you experienced during the fight, then simply share them with your partner.

This is not the time to explain why you felt them or what triggered them. Just let your partner know what feelings were bubbling inside you. For example, you might have felt angry, resentful, frustrated, or indignant during the fight. You might also have experienced feelings like sadness, hurt, or fear. Did you feel overwhelmed, ashamed, guilty, or remorseful? Perhaps, even lonely, unloved, disliked, or abandoned? Be as comprehensive as you can. Give your partner a complete picture of the feelings you experienced. Perhaps this softens the atmosphere just a bit.

Then, it's your partner's turn to share.

## Step Two: Describing Your Movie

This step asks each of you to share your story. To describe the movie you carry inside.

*Speaker:* Describe your memory of what happened, focusing on what you recall. Only share what *you* heard, what *you* saw, how *you* felt. Don't make the case for your movie being true but instead share it as your truth. Don't talk about what you think your partner meant or intended, but rather share your movie, paint your picture. Use descriptive, non-blaming language. Let your partner in on your experience.

*Listener:* After listening to your partner, try to summarize their experience—their reality, their movie. You're not here to defend yourself or be a critic. You're here to witness and reflect their story. To let them know you really see their movie and understand their experience. Now step forward and validate their reality. Just as in the Gottman-Rapoport exercise, validation doesn't mean you agree with their story or that you're invalidating your own experience. It's not about that. It's simply about you being present with your partner's experience and recognizing it as their reality.

Before switching roles, confirm that your partner feels their reality has been seen, heard, and validated.

Now, switch roles. Same process. Same procedure.

When done well, the toxicity of the fight will have been at least partially neutralized.

## Step Three: Identifying Your Triggers

This step is somewhat a leap of faith. You're asked to return to the fight and identify what triggered you. Describe the specific moments during the fight that were emotionally challenging, then explore why those moments were so upsetting.

Next, scan your life history. Look for times in the past when you experienced similar triggering moments. Open those files. Permit yourself to remember what you experienced and how you felt. Now breathe a bit. Can you share them, or even some of them, with your partner? This can be a vulnerable moment. Share what you're comfortable revealing. Don't feel obliged to go to places that don't feel safe. Common triggers include feelings like, *I felt judged, threatened, unsafe, criticized, lonely, or powerless.* These are just a few; the list is endless.

Now, back to your partner. After hearing your partner's triggering experience and their history with that feeling, can you, once again, validate their experience? Did you allow their trigger story to touch you? Could you visualize them in that situation? Did it open compassion within you? Validation for this kind of sharing, after this level of vulnerability, is crucial; it begins to establish you as a safe person for them.

Now it's time to switch roles and for your opportunity to explore and share.

## Step Four: Taking Some Responsibility

This step introduces another opportunity to soften the fight and create more connection. Here, you're each asked to take a counterintuitive step: to admit that you were part of the problem and to take some degree of responsibility for the fight. By dropping the cloak of defensiveness and owning your part, you breathe fresh air into a stagnant atmosphere. I'm not suggesting you need to take full responsibility for the fight, just step up and own part of it. As you do so, you lift that amount of weight off your partner's shoulders. They feel less blamed. Not quite so implicated. Their load lightens.

Here are some themes you might consider:

"I just wasn't my best self during that fight. These aren't excuses… just explanations that I didn't fully realize at the time."

"I've been feeling overwhelmed, emotionally depleted, sensitive, critical, or irritable."

> "As I go through the day, I've had a chip on my shoulder and have felt insecure or stressed."
>
> "As I look back, I realize that I've been emotionally distant, haven't spent time with you, haven't been a good listener, and just wanted to be alone. I've been really overwhelmed."
>
> No excuses, just admitting and owning.
>
> Now, complete the loop by offering an apology: "I'm sorry, you didn't deserve that, it's on me. I'm especially sorry for how this became part of the fight. I lashed out at you when all you did was ask a question. Can you accept my apology?"
>
> Once again, time to switch roles.
>
> **Step Five: Designing a Constructive Plan**
>
> Now, after completing the first four steps you're in a much better position to consider the future. Think about what you could do differently and what you would like your partner to do differently when a similar issue arises in the future. What would help you avoid falling into a fight or allow you to keep it respectful and manageable?
>
> Lead off by offering what you could do differently. Then make a a similar request of your partner.
>
> Switch roles and ask your partner to share their views too.
>
> Then discuss and agree on a game plan to try in the future.
>
> Practice this exercise using a real but not too emotionally loaded topic.

# The Grip of Gridlock

As you work to build a relationship that is sustainable, you must develop the skill of addressing those issues that have the greatest likelihood of not just frustrating you, but of dividing you.

All relationships have issues. About thirty percent of couples' problems are "solvable." When you address them directly, with the intent of coming up with a solution that works for both of you, there's a good chance

## Attunement: From Avoiding to Addressing Issues

you'll get there. These problems are part of everyday living. They are sometimes annoying but fundamentally resolvable. The solution is often simply a matter of discussing and compromising on the issue at hand. The focus is usually on "what" needs to be done, "who" will do the task, "how" it will be done, or "when" it's to be completed. It's not that solvable problems are easy; it's more that both of you approach them with an air of cooperation or "let's work it out." Neither of you come to the table with a closed mind or determination that you're going to "win" this one. As you might have already discovered, in the world of intimate relationships, "winning" is the most direct path to "losing." Over time, the loss of connection is the cost.

The remaining seventy percent of couples' problems are chronic and persistent. They're labeled "perpetual" problems. These issues are a matter of more concern. In and of themselves, they don't necessarily threaten the future of your relationship. They can't be "solved" because they're reflective of basic differences between you. Basic differences of personality, lifestyle preferences, wants, wishes, or needs. How you like to spend your leisure time, your work-life balance, how you view finances, the importance of affection and sex, the kids' education, the centrality of the extended family, and on and on. What makes them persistent is your differentness. As long as you can talk about them with respect and caring, work to meet both of your needs, and compromise with one another, they're manageable—never really resolved but not relationship threatening.

But a subgroup of these perpetual problems may pose a more serious threat to your relationship. When you lose the ability to discuss your feelings and needs around any of these issues, when attempts to discuss them result in tension, fights, or cutoffs, they're at risk of transforming into a more pernicious threat. When in addition to being areas of differentness, you find yourselves at an impasse over them, warning sirens sound. They're at risk of becoming "gridlocked."

And gridlocked issues have the potential to create emotional distance, escalating conflict, bitterness, and resentment. You have the same fight over and over. You become more and more entrenched in your positions. Neither one of you feels you can compromise. It devolves into a clear win-lose dynamic. Respect wanes (Gottman and Gottman 2024). It's from this emerging place of polarization that a downward spiral gains momentum.

Then, even when you do take the risk of trying once again, it goes poorly. There's no openness or receptivity between you and your partner. Well-intentioned words or gestures fall to the wayside and small, even unintended, words, gestures, or tones are interpreted as adversarial or hostile. You begin to vilify one another, at first internally, then eventually externally. You experience your partner not only as stubborn but also as selfish or narcissistic. Hope fades.

While on the surface the topic of your dispute might not seem to warrant such an intense struggle, there's more to it than meets the eye. Any topic has the potential to become gridlocked. It's not about the subject, it's about how strongly you both feel about that issue and how difficult it is to have an open, respectful conversation about it. Gridlocked issues are typically embedded in deeper issues. They're about unfulfilled dreams, or core, value-based ideas deep within you. While you may not be exactly clear why you feel so strongly about the issue, or why you're so unyielding in your position, you are clear that you can bend no further. And, as both of you arrive at that juncture, the knot tightens.

As polarizing, frustrating, and demoralizing as gridlock can be, there is hope. Not so much in immediately untying the knot, but in seeing it, studying it, and understanding it. The path to dealing with gridlock is for you and your partner to work through it, not try to go around it.

Given all you've been through and are still going through in the aftermath of betrayal, learning to deal with gridlock in an open, healthy, respectful manner is a required skill. The next exercise will provide a map. The goal of this exercise is to shift from the polarization and stuckness of gridlock back to respect for your differentness and a collaborative mindset. This is how happily connected partners deal with gridlock. After developing this, you'll be more successful in developing a sustainable, win-win compromise on the issue.

As you work on a gridlocked issue, it's helpful to approach it with the awareness that there's something about this particular topic that is making it impossible for either of you to just give in. Starting with a sense of interest and curiosity is the best way to begin. You know that you're stuck in an impasse. You realize the outcome of this issue is really important to you but compromising feels out of the question. You don't quite see why your partner couldn't be more agreeable, or flexible—just this one time. This is the nature of gridlock.

> ### Exercise: **Dreams Within Conflict**
>
> *This exercise is for both of you.*
>
> In this intervention, you'll be asked to step back from the impasse, stop pulling on the rope, and permit the knot to loosen just a bit. The focus will be on more fully understanding why your position and the position of your partner are so strong. What emotional needs are underlying those positions? What core values are fueling them (Gottman and Gottman 2024)? As you're both able to more clearly understand the "why" of the depth of your needs, as well as those of your partner, the knot will loosen. You'll realize your partner wasn't just being stubborn or selfish. You'll recognize they were fighting for some deeply held need founded in a value.
>
> For example, you might be gridlocked over money. What to save, what to spend? When to save, when to spend? How to save, how to spend? While this may have always felt like a perpetual issue for you, an area of fundamentally different opinions, it feels different now. It's more intense. You're not able to work it out. You can't even talk about it without a familiar fight. It's like being pulled into a play you've repeated over and over. You both know your lines as well as your partner's. They're painful to repeat but you do so anyway. Resolution seems impossible. Even the idea of compromise feels unattainable. It would be a lose-lose.
>
> The purpose of this exercise is to understand why this issue has become so, so important. It's no longer about differing preferences; it's about something essential. Maybe even a deal breaker. For example, gridlock over a topic like money sometimes has its roots in a struggle over saving or stability vs. spending and living life now. For you, it may be about your desire to give your children the life you wish you had when you were young. For your partner, it might be about saving for education so the children have the opportunity to create whatever life they dream of for themselves. The key to

loosening the knot is the recognition of the depth of the love you both feel for your children. You're both pushing to act in their best interests. You're driven by a similar desire...to do what's best for them. From this perspective, you're actually on the same team. The problem is that you have different ideas about what that looks like. From this place of genuine caring and concern for your children, real conversation becomes possible.

This realization doesn't resolve the problem, but it does soften the gridlock. This exercise is just about truly understanding your own and your partner's position on this gridlocked issue. On gridlocked topics, understanding comes before problem-solving. Until you clearly see and appreciate the value-based depth of both positions, there's no basis for a genuine compromise conversation.

## Preparation for the Exercise

This is another Speaker-Listener exercise. It may be important to consider who should start as the Speaker and who should start as the Listener. Both roles have some important guidelines. Be sure you're both able to meet these requirements.

- Identify three topics that feel like gridlock. Remember, it's not really about the topic, it's about how stuck you are over it.

- Explore what makes each topic so important to you.

- Talk with your partner and agree to a time to begin this exercise.

## Doing the Exercise

Look at your lists and select a topic to begin with.

*Check in with yourself.* Are you calm enough, open enough, and curious enough about your partner's position to do this exercise? Remember it's about understanding, not problem-solving. That comes later.

*The Speaker's role* is to simply try to describe your position on this issue. Share what you think and how you feel. Let you partner know what it means to you and why it's so important to you without trying to convince them to agree with you.

*The Listener's role* is to interview your partner to help them explore or explain their views on the issue. This role can be difficult to truly enter. Please use the following questions to guide the conversation. You can ask additional follow-up questions to further explore your partner's feelings and needs, but don't make it about you. Don't dispute or challenge their position; just help them explore their position. Your job is to make your partner feel comfortable exploring and sharing their views with you on a difficult issue. Try to suspend judgement as your partner speaks. Help them feel that you're interested in what they think, feel and need. Perhaps ask the questions like a good friend would. Be patient and curious. Try to keep your opinions, thoughts, or needs out of this interaction. You'll have the chance to share your views when you're the Speaker.

## *Questions to Guide the Interaction*

Begin here with the Listener asking the Speaker these questions:

- What do you believe about this issue? Can you describe any value it's connected to? What does it mean to you?

- How is this influenced by your past? How is it related to your childhood, to time with your family, other relationships, or life experiences?

- I know this is important to you, but why is it *this* important to you?

- As you think about this issue, what are your strongest feelings?

- What is your ideal dream on this issue?

- So, what is the need or purpose under this dream?
- What is your greatest fear if this need is never met?

As the Speaker, is there anything you would like to add so your partner can understand more about your position? This is not yet the time for problem-solving. (That's in the next exercise.)

As the Listener, briefly summarize what you now understand about your partner's position. This is not yet the time to problem-solve or advocate for your position.

The next step is to change roles and allow the Listener to become the Speaker. Are you ready to begin the second part or would either of you like a break?

Remember that as the Speaker, your job is to explore why this issue is so important to you. What need or value is it connected to? It's not to rebut your partner's position. Practice the Dreams Within Conflict exercise using a real but not too emotionally loaded topic.

At the end of this exercise, you will have a better understanding of *why* this issue became gridlocked. You see how it's connected to core values that need to be honored. Rather than seeing your partner as stubborn, you realize they were just trying to honor a deeply held value or belief. Even if it didn't go smoothly the whole time, take heart in any progress you did make. The negative power of gridlock is difficult to break. You may need to do this exercise more than once on entrenched issues.

## Crafting a Compromise

Now, from a place of understanding and compassion, negotiating a compromise is more possible. You're now in the position to talk as friends, both of you wanting the other to be pleased with the compromise you craft. You're in collaborative rather than adversarial positions.

The mindset you bring to this exercise is critical. Make it your goal to emerge with an agreement that feels right to both of you. Rather than insisting on a specific concession, begin by looking for

## Attunement: From Avoiding to Addressing Issues

> common ground. Try to notice aspects of your partner's needs that might fit with your core needs. Work to honor your needs as well as those of your partner. Adopt a win-win perspective. "Yes, I want what I want, but not at your expense."
>
> A final point to consider is to approach this exercise realizing that a partial or temporary compromise may be the prudent way to begin. Don't start seeking a solution you'll live with for the rest of your life. Start with something that represents a positive step that you'll revisit later.

---

### Exercise: **Compromise Ovals**

*This exercise is for both of you.*

Select a topic that's important but that doesn't feel too entrenched. If you both now feel understood on the topic you addressed in the Dreams Within Conflict exercise, you might use that same topic.

Before beginning this exercise, be sure both of you have a notebook or sheet of paper and a pencil on which you'll draw a large donut or bagel. You'll be asked to enter your core needs in the center circle, then fill in the larger circle with your areas of flexibility. Afterward, you will ask each other questions about what you've written and establish a compromise agreement.

*Step one.* Begin by stepping back. Take a few minutes to give serious consideration to what you need from this compromise to feel good about the agreement. Be honest with yourself. These are your non-negotiables: don't be too sacrificial or betray your needs. Don't give up something that's really important to you. On the other hand, don't ask for the moon.

Write these core needs in the center circle.

*Step two.* Now that you've defined what you need, shift your attention to what you can be flexible about. What can you do or give up to meet your partner's core needs without betraying yourself?

List all the ways you can stretch or flex without feeling resentful. This is the time to be expansive and creative. It's an opportunity to step outside of yourself and let your partner know that you care about them and their needs.

The motto is simple: "I want what I want, and I want you to have what you want." Enter these ideas in the larger circle.

*Step three.* Now, share your lists with your partner. Simply read what you came up with. Don't discuss or negotiate quite yet. Let the words you heard from your partner sink in. Be sure you're hearing their core needs, but be equally certain you're taking in all the ways they're willing to be flexible. This injects positivity into the atmosphere as you prepare to have a compromise conversation.

*Step four.* Please use the following questions as a guide to discussing the issue and crafting a compromise. View this as your initial effort to create a path. What you come up with today might be considered a partial or temporary compromise. Define it and try it out for a week or two. Schedule a time to revisit your agreement and make any changes indicated.

## Compromise Questions

Use these questions to guide you. Have a conversation rather than using the Speaker-Listener approach.

1. Help me understand why the things in your inner circle are so crucial to you. What do they mean to you?

2. Say more about your areas of flexibility. What can you stretch on to support my needs?

3. What do we have in common? What do you see as our common goals? Be as descriptive as possible.

4. What do we agree about? Be specific.

5. What feelings do we have in common?

> 6. What steps can we take to accomplish these goals? Define each step.
>
> *Step five.* Write out a compromise agreement you'll live by this week. Be specific about the conditions and set a time to revisit it in a week.
>
> Practice the Compromise Ovals exercise using a real but not too emotionally loaded topic. For example, finding time to talk and connect with each other on a more regular basis; spending twenty minutes with each other, without screens, after you get the kids to bed; or getting the kids to bed earlier might be part of this agreement. Alternatively, you might opt to create and protect a longer period of time together two or three times a week. Creating and protecting couple's time is an essential component of intimate connection.

Mastering these four skills will permit you to address rather than avoid important relationship issues. Your willingness to lean into, rather than away from, tough issues will buffer your relationship from unexpected crises.

# In Closing

The focus of this chapter was to help you to move toward your partner and away from avoidance. Avoidance creates disconnect...distance. When you establish a default setting of avoidance, you grow apart. It's the opposite of being attuned. You now have the tools to lean in. You now know how to stay present and turn toward your partner, even on issues of disagreement and especially in moments of disconnect. You are now beginning to operate on the idea that while sharing your inner thoughts and feelings carries a certain vulnerability, it's riskier to not share them.

CHAPTER 8

# Attunement: Revitalizing Your Friendship

In the last chapter, you crossed the bridge from avoiding to addressing areas of concern. You've developed the skills required to turn toward and address difficult issues in a caring, respectful fashion. As is true with all new skills, they take practice.

## Creating the Conditions of Connection

Now let's focus on revitalizing your friendship. The fabric of your bond has been torn—it's time to work on it. The exercises and skills here are for both of you.

Friendship begins with a sense of presence. It involves being interested and curious about the other and bringing your authentic self to the encounter. At the most basic level, friendship is about *being* known and *feeling* known. It's about a real lived relationship, not just fantasy and imagination. In a friendship, you ask questions and share stories that reveal your inner self. You make visible your values, ethics, and beliefs. You're open to hearing and trying to understand each other.

It's hard to find a person you can truly be yourself with. As partners who have been through so much together, your life is not a new canvas. You've painted many experiences on it. You've traversed real life together. The highs and the lows. The joys as well as the sorrows. Can you approach your relationship again, with new eyes, fresh ears, and an open heart? There's one additional ingredient to consider: the investment of time. Engaged time is required to create friendship.

# The Best of Us

Can you recall the early days of your relationship? Not just the facts of when you met or where you met but more importantly *who* you met? What did you notice? What was that initial attraction? What were you drawn to? Beyond that, how did you decide to see each other again? You carry within you a story of your beginning. The actual experience of your journey from first encounter to commitment. You may have been young or impulsive, perhaps even needy or insecure. But there was a certain wisdom that was your guide. You chose one another for some good reasons. There was something compelling about your togetherness.

## *The Best of Us: The Story of Us*

In addition to the physical attraction, the fun, the "easy to be together" themes, as you spent more time together, what did you begin to learn about each other? What qualities or characteristics made an impression? What stood out? *He was funny…she was nice. We could talk all night. He was relaxed and comfortable. Attentive and intense. Deep and dark. She was light and happy. Energetic and open. Social and sexy.*

Yes, there's a love story of your beginning. Actually, two stories, the one you carry and the one that resides in your partner. In some ways, they're similar. In others, they may be different. It's fair to say that most beginnings are beautiful. And even if troubled, there were beautiful moments.

As you moved forward, when did it occur to you that this relationship might have a future? That there was more to it than the fun and excitement?

How did you move from dating to dedicated? Did trust come easily or was it a hard-won accomplishment?

Did commitment simply emerge or did you actually talk about it? Did you fight about it? Did you struggle with boundaries?

This is not to say that there may not have been issues too. There were times you may have clashed or felt moments of disappointment and disconnect. Instances you entertained doubts about a future together. If there were breakups, you came back together again. In real time, you made a choice. You committed.

Give yourself the gift of revisiting your stories. Those beginnings, times of dreams and hope, may hold a key to your future. Buried within are moments of connection.

Over time, disappointment, loneliness, resentment, and most powerfully, betrayal rewrote the story of your beginning. The infidelity that brought you to this place has colored your memories. Your story now contains chapters on betrayal and loss, broken trust and violated commitment. Yes, trust and commitment, those words that once offered safety and certainty, have now been redefined. You can no longer give them freely. They must be earned. And yet, there remain, early in your relationship, memories of the lived experiences that were real and compelling. And now, as you consider committing to your partner once again, those memories can offer another kind of comfort. What you once experienced, who you once were, still resonates within.

So turn back the clock to those early times. Do it as a gift to yourself, your partner, and your relationship. Enjoy them. Just to be clear, accessing those memories doesn't guarantee a positive future. They're not meant to convince you to stay in a situation that's not right for you. There's still work to be done to be sure this relationship offers what you need. Is your partner the person you will choose again?

## Exercise: Back to the Beginning

*This exercise is for both partners.*

**Part 1:** Revisit and journal about the story of your relationship: your experience of the life you created and lived from the beginning to the betrayal. Use these questions as a guide as you revisit your story. The next step will be to share this with your partner:

- What was the initial attraction?
- As you spent more time together and got to know each other better, what pulled you even closer?
- Were there things that worried you?

- What about trust? Was it just naturally there or did you need to work on it?
- Were there moments when trust was broken?
- Did you address or avoid it? Did you resolve anything or simply try to move past it?
- How did you decide to commit to this relationship and a life together?
- Over time, what qualities in your partner were most important to you?
- When things were going well, what made the relationship work for you?
- What were the most powerful moments, the most special times of connection for you?
- When things were difficult, what were your frustrations/concerns?
- What wants, wishes, needs went unmet?
- How did you deal with them?

**Part 2:** Share your story with your partner. Your experience of the relationship from the beginnings to the betrayal. As you move into this step of sharing your story, use the skills you learned earlier in *Healing the Trauma of Infidelity*.

## Exercise: Communication Skills for the Conversation

*This exercise is for both partners.*

- Before beginning…settle yourselves. Calm your nervous systems.

- Recognize there are two stories. Both have validity and both need to be heard.

- When you're listening to your partner's story, calm your rebuttal brain. Try to understand and see it from their point of view.

- Share your story as your truth, your experience. It's the story that resides within you.

- Speak from the perspective of how you felt, what you experienced, what you remember.

- Minimize comments about what your partner did or said. Don't mention your partner's intent.

- When listening, don't contest the "truth" of any part of your partner's story.

- When you feel the need to correct or contest…breathe.

- As you listen, do you notice a bit of compassion for your partner?

- Can you see and validate your partner's experience? You don't need to agree with them to validate their experience.

# The Bond and the Betrayal

At one time, you chose your partner over all others. You saw something special in them. It wasn't just looks, intelligence, ambition, or social standing…you saw a person you could entrust your life to. A person you could build a life with. You saw a person of character. Someone you admired. You loved their kindness, their depth, their presence. You knew them to their core: they'd be a great partner in good times and bad, a dedicated parent, someone you could lean on and trust with everything.

## Attunement: Revitalizing Your Friendship

*And then the betrayal.* The person you chose, the person you knew, the person you committed to could never do that. It was devastating and disorienting.

The pain of the betrayal and the need to protect yourself from future hurt quite naturally lead you to see your partner through different eyes. Now, with the issues you've addressed and the strengths you've developed...*who do you see now when you look at your partner?* Do you see a person who has owned their failings, felt your pain, and expressed genuine remorse? Has that remorse turned into action? Is your partner doing their own work? Are they dedicated to being there with you and healing your hurts? Or are they merely waiting for you to come around? These are important questions.

---

### Exercise: **Who are You?**

*This exercise is for both of you.*

This exercise invites you to rethink how you see your partner.

1. List the key personal traits in your partner that led you to choose them. Kindness, caring, energy, and the like. Do you still see those qualities in them? Do they show them with you?

2. Think of times when your partner was there for you and displayed each of these qualities. Recall how you felt in those moments. Do you still see evidence of them?

This exercise is a simple way of remembering positive feelings about your partner. Do they still reside within you, even if they're hidden or not so frequently revealed?

The next step is to share these positive traits with your partner. Now, find a quiet moment to share and let them know what you valued and appreciated.

# Friendship and Attunement

Learning to focus on and attune to your partner's feelings and experiences is an important skill to master as you begin to rebuild your friendship. Here are a few ideas to work on:

*Prepare yourself to listen.* As simple as this sounds, it's a difficult skill to master. Strive to get comfortable with the idea of temporarily putting your thoughts on the back burner and truly be interested in your partner's experience.

*Enter their world.* Again, simple but difficult! Try to put yourself in their shoes. Hear their words and be cognizant of emotions that may reside within. Learn to ask questions that invite them to share more and more of their deeper feelings and needs.

*Ask open-ended questions.* These are questions that can't be answered with a simple yes or no response. They invite more thought and exploration. For example:

- "What are your deepest feelings and needs about this?"
- "What do you wish for regarding this issue?"
- "Can you tell me a story of when you felt something similar in the past?"
- "Can you tell me what makes this so powerful to you?"
- "What do you really need me to understand right now?"

*Express empathy and understanding.* In additional to being heard, it's important for your partner to feel that their words, feelings, and needs matter to you. That you're moved by their experience. The following phrases convey caring and empathy:

- "I'd feel that way too if that happened to me."
- "I wish I would have been there with you."

- "That would have upset me too."
- "When you're hurting that much, I want to help."
- "That really makes sense."
- "You're right."
- "I really admire how you handled that impossible situation."

Attunement is a specific type of presence that emphasizes emotional connection and empathic engagement. It leaves your partner feeling they're not alone and that you value and care for them.

# Dealing with Drift: Making Time for Us

Drift is part of relational living. No matter how close you are, no matter how committed you feel, there are moments when you lose contact. You're captured by work, the kids, or your hobbies. At times you just need to be alone. This sort of drift occurs in the best of relationships. It can be likened to the loss of gravitational pull. In happy, stable relationships, moments or periods of drift lead to corrective action. One of you will notice that you feel a bit disconnected or that your partner seems preoccupied or distant. So you mention it. You reach for them and they engage and respond. You might use an "I miss you" approach. You move closer without much effort. You address it while still under the influence of gravitational pull.

In other cases, the scenario isn't quite so benign. You've drifted further apart. Your lessening connection isn't noticed as quickly. And by the time you do see it, one or both of you may have floated beyond the influence of gravitational pull. Your sense of connection has weakened. In this situation, it doesn't go as smoothly. Negative emotions, low interest, or lack of motivation now complicate the likelihood of a simple, natural corrective action. Rather than finding words for an "I miss you" approach, you find yourself starting with a "where the hell have you been" attitude. (More on this in the next chapter.)

# Prioritize Your Relationship

So, what's the best preventative strategy? It's simple. Start by making time together a priority as well as a pattern. Over time, this can make a real difference.

### *Create a Ritual for a Daily Emotional Check-In*

In the wake of infidelity and the pain of knowing that your partner chose someone else, you now need the experience of your partner choosing you, over and over.

A daily emotional check-in demonstrates that you're on your partner's mind and that what you're feeling matters to them. This kind of time together is different than talking about work or the kids. It's not just watching a movie or working in the garden together. It's more personal. (By the way, there's a place for all of those things too.)

The ritual you create should be tailored to meet your specific needs. A question like "How was your day?" may morph into "What are you feeling right now?" Additional questions might be as direct as "Did you struggle with anything about my affair today?" or as general as "What was your high and low of the day?" "What do you need right now?" or "How would you like to spend time together tonight?" might hit the spot. Sharing comments like "I missed you today," or "I'm sorry I couldn't call, but you were on my mind" make a difference. Conveying the spirit of "I miss you and you matter to me" is what counts.

Begin by finding the right moments to spend this time together. While this may sound superficial, the idea of creating predictable, repeatable time together is no small matter. And it's not just repeatable time, but it's also quality time. Time when you have the energy to be present, engaged and awake.

Mornings work well for some couples while the end of the workday is preferable to others. While late evening works for some couples, beware of late hours. The goal is to give your partner the best of you. Talking when either one of you is exhausted or depleted may miss the mark. Whenever you have your conversation, be mindful of your energy levels, the kids, job responsibilities, activities, and the myriad of things that compete for your time. Make sure the television is off and screens are down. Offer the gift of a few minutes of your undivided attention. Consider, too, starting with a hug and sharing an appreciation. This small connection done regularly makes a difference.

After a week, discuss your experience of the talks. Adjust as needed.

## *My Go-To Person*

In addition to the emotional check-in, conversations about your experience of the day matter too. An important part of friendship is developing the sense that "You're my go-to person. You're the person I turn to when I want to share my thoughts and feelings with someone. When I have something to share, I naturally go to you."

Here's a simple practice to adopt. At dinner, or sometime later in the day, take a few minutes to put into words your "high and low" of the day. Think about this as recalling and sharing a moment in the day that evoked a positive emotion and another moment that called forth a negative emotion. If you're naturally emotionally expressive, this will be easy. If being emotionally dismissive is your style, it may feel awkward and take a bit of work, but it's an attainable skill.

# Opportunity Knocks: Making Bids and Turning Toward Bids

In the flow of everyday living, nothing is more important than feeling close. How do you try to achieve that closeness? You make a *bid*. A bid is any word or action you make in hopes of creating a moment of connection (Gottman and DeClaire 2001). While bids can be subtle, indirect or even irritable, it's important to recognize that they're a way of reaching out to you. As a partner, your task is to be aware, sensitive and responsive to even hidden bids. You need to (1) notice, (2) receive, and (3) respond to your partner reaching out for you.

When your partner enters the room and plops down beside you on the couch with a sigh, tune in; that was a bid. *Notice* they entered the room and chose to sit by you, *receive* the bid, and understand the wish behind *the plop and sigh* (they want a moment of connection), and *respond* with something like "What's up honey? Anything on your mind?" For extra credit, you might start with something like "Nice to see you, glad you're here." If you're really aware, when you see them enter the room, you might pat the couch next to you and invite them to join you.

Just remember, a bid is a request for emotional engagement, perhaps direct or maybe thinly veiled. But in either case, it is a request for connection. Why not just always be direct? The answer is that making a bid, asking for engagement, comes with a risk. The risk of rejection. You feel vulnerable.

When I reach for you, you have three choices. You can turn toward my bid as described in the "plop and sigh" example regarding the couch. That would be great. And when you take that option, all is well. On the other hand, you could turn away by simply saying or doing nothing. Not acknowledging my presence. In that case, I have choices to consider. I can quietly take it as rejection and feel uncared for. Or, perhaps I'll calmly persist by expressing the story behind the sigh: "Even though we've been home all day, I feel like I haven't even seen you. I miss you. Can we turn off the television and hang out together?" On the other hand, if silence is a familiar response, I might add a zinger such as "Hello, earth to space cadet…do you read me?" or with even more hurt and frustration: "Do you even care how I feel?"

Your other option would be turning against, a more aggressive response to the "plop and sigh" entry. You might begin with "Can't you see I'm watching the game? Get some manners!" You might escalate with "Show a bit of respect! It's all about you, isn't it? You're just like your mother!" In an even more reactive moment, the words "I don't know why I put up with this abuse. I never should have married you in the first place!" can flow too easily.

Bids sometimes carry an emotional loading, a sensitivity to rejection. Reactive moments are not far away. Bids come in all shapes and sizes. A bid can take the form of a question, an invitation, or even a gesture:

## Attunement: Revitalizing Your Friendship

Questions: "Do you have a minute?"; "What do you think about the new movie, the election, your mom's birthday?"; "Are you OK?"; "How are you feeling?"

Invitations: "Would you like to go for a walk?"; "The weekend is almost here, what would you like to do?"; "Can we make some time together?"

Gestures: Pointing to a bird in the backyard, touching your shoulder as you pass in the hallway, making a pouty facial expression.

Try to respond to your partner's bids by turning toward. That tells your partner "You matter to me, your experience touches me, and how you feel is important." It requires just three steps: (1) notice, (2) receive, and (3) respond.

*Notice.* This first step is noticing. For some, it's easy—it's how they move through life. They look around, pay attention to who is around them, and what is happening around them. For others, it takes effort. Whatever your natural style, make awareness of your partner a priority. You might wonder, *Is he upstairs with the kids?*; *Is she outside with the dog?*; *Is he taking a nap?*; *Is she talking to her mom?* No need for a tracking device, but practice being curious about your partner.

*Receive.* This step is more specific than the general idea of noticing. Here, you're being asked to develop a specific attentiveness to what your partner is doing and saying as well as what it means. What message is being sent by your partner? What are they wanting you to receive and understand? Add context to the mix. What issues and responsibilities are on their plate? What stressors are in their life? Did they sleep well last night? What is their facial expression telling you? This skill starts with attentiveness. Look at your partner with curiosity, not judgment.

*Respond.* Now let's look at how you respond, what you do or say. Based on what you've noticed, received, and now understand, you may be able to see your partner's point of view. You may recognize their positive intention. Remember you have three basic choices: you either turn toward, turn away, or turn against. Turning toward is more common when you're in a positive space with one another. You receive your partner's bid and realize they're seeking connection.

When you're not feeling so positive about the relationship, it's difficult to respond well. You're more likely to turn away or turn against. These responses add to the negativity.

## Small Moments, Large Results

Happy couples experience a lot of positivity in their daily interactions. Not all of these moments are intense, emotional experiences. In fact, many of them are small, mundane experiences. What they represent, however, is a consistent, positive-leaning turning toward attitude.

One of the most impactful of these small moments is referred to as "fondness and admiration" (Gottman and Gottman 2024). Happy couples populate the atmosphere with positive comments about one another. Some are as basic as thanking one another for a task, event, or responsibility they complete. Loading the dishwasher, taking the trash out, making sure the kids are out of bed, putting the kids to bed, making coffee in the morning… small but significant. Being appreciated for what you do is important.

Another more personal variety of appreciation is valuing your partner for who they are. Now you're talking about the personal qualities of your partner that make them special to you. Even here, some qualities are more personal than others. Hearing that you appreciate your partner's dependability is nice. Comments about their kindness, generosity, or humor are even better. When you tell them you love their smile, or are drawn to their energy, their heart warms. Sharing that you find them attractive, or feel lucky to have them in your life, really catches their attention.

One convenient method for bringing these principles into play in everyday life is called "seeing, sending, receiving."

## Attunement: Revitalizing Your Friendship

### *Seeing, Sending, Receiving*

Begin with the simple act of *seeing,* of being mindful of the actions, words, and personal qualities of your partner that you value. Things they do, moments you observe that touch you. Things that make them appealing to you.

The next step is to *send* this awareness to them. Find words, actions or gestures that express your appreciation to your partner. There's a bit of skill involved in this step. The challenge is to share your appreciations at a time, in a manner, and in a language your partner is likely to receive. This is back to the "intent is not the same as impact" axiom. Paying attention to your timing and delivery matters.

The final piece of the process, *receiving,* is to be sure the message sent is the message received. Being mindful and expressing appreciation is of little value until it's received. At times, it's obvious. At others, less so. Following up with "Hey honey. I want to make sure I said this clearly enough…I really love your kindness" (or "…am drawn to your energy" or "…find you attractive") can make a difference.

By the way, there may be moments when your partner just isn't in a place to receive your appreciation. In those moments, stick with the spirit you had when you sent it. Don't revert to "You never appreciate anything," or "Why am I the only one who's trying?" An appreciation offered with love doesn't call for an argument. Let it stand on its own merits.

## Rituals of Connection

As you're feeling more valued and connected, perhaps life is beginning to brighten. You may notice more positive feelings. There's sometimes a bit of a bounce in your step. The heaviness that once engulfed you may be losing its power. Now is the time to create patterns of living that support the gains you've made. A time to develop ways of going through daily living that help you feel connected (Gottman and Gottman 2024). A time to create a flow that makes your closeness sustainable.

These rituals can be large or small. They're patterns that keep you leaning in. They naturally support turning toward and being present.

## *Transitions*

The beauty of transition rituals is that they often generate a big return on a small amount of time. While there are many moments of transition in daily living, here are four that offer real opportunity:

1. When you see your partner for the first time after waking, what happens? What would the camera notice? Do you talk, touch, or silently trudge past one another?

2. What's the pattern when one of you leaves the house or heads to their office to work? Is there an embrace and positive send off? Or do you separate without a glance?

3. What's the ritual when you're both finally home after being apart for the day? This may be the most important of the routine transitions of daily living because it sets the emotional tone for the evening.

4. What's your bedtime routine? Do you end the day with a moment of connection, or is it a rejecting or neglecting moment that ends the day? Falling asleep with a sense of gratitude instead of resentment or loneliness contributes to the quality of your sleep.

Here are a few more moments to consider ritualizing:

*Keeping close when apart.* When you're away from each other for a significant amount of time, create a daily pattern to connect. Call or text just to let your partner know you were thinking about them.

*Mutually enjoyable activity.* Look for gaps in your schedule or times you can clear to spend time together doing something you both naturally enjoy. Set a schedule to do these activities on a regular basis. Without the schedule, well-intended plans seem to fall by the wayside. It could be as simple as a midweek lunch, or an after-dinner walk. Making it regular and something you both look forward to is the key.

*Affection.* Add moments of affection to the flow of everyday living. How long is your typical hug? Three seconds, maybe four? Bump it to twenty seconds and notice the difference.

*Emotional Check-In* or *My Go-To Person conversations.* Establish the pattern of seeking and sharing with one another on a regular basis.

*Date night.* Prioritizing romantic time together, away from the responsibilities and stress of family life, is important. Put in the time and energy required to create a getaway. It could be a walk in the park and a picnic, a quiet dinner, or maybe even a noisy dinner. Make it something that fits what you need at that moment in time. There may be times when it's more comfortable to have an activity to focus on such as a movie or a play. At others, a more intimate setting may be called for. A time when you can relax and just attend to each other.

In some moments, you may want to plan the activity, at others it may be important to have your partner surprise you. Perhaps a conversation and a joint decision works at other times. The key is to make it part of your pattern (Gottman et al., 2008).

# In Closing

In this chapter, you have created the foundation of friendship. Secure in the experience that your feelings and needs matter, and with trust growing, you're now more comfortable leaning in. You were able to revisit your history and the beauty that was once there. You re-experienced some of the power of your early bond and remembered life experiences that drew you close. You worked on bids and turning toward, fondness and admiration, and rituals of connection.

CHAPTER 9

# The Path to Infidelity

The challenging work of this chapter is only possible after you've become skilled at self-regulation and worked on your communication skills. Progress in the atonement and attunement chapters is also helpful.

Here, the focus shifts to exploring how betrayal entered your relationship. As the Hurt Partner, you need a clearer sense of what happened. This understanding will guide you in creating a relationship that is not susceptible to future betrayals. You can't go there again! You won't go there again! In this regard, your partner's work is to identify and describe what happened and how they crossed the line to betrayal. It's part of the basis for creating a new, quake-proof foundation.

For you, the Involved Partner, this chapter shifts to your internal experience. The themes, patterns, and experiences described here are intended to highlight areas for you to explore. Some will ring true for you. Others may miss the mark. This chapter is about seeking understanding of the betrayal. The work is to bring clarity and understanding to what happened. It's not about justification, blame, or condemnation. You're invited to step out of self-deceit and away from self-justification. These attitudes permitted you to violate a boundary you otherwise would not have crossed. It's especially important that you don't blame your partner for your actions. The behavior is yours to own. This isn't easy work. It takes courage. It's related to your decision, your conviction, to now do the right thing.

While it's commonly assumed that affairs are primarily about seeking sex, in many situations, loneliness and the loss of closeness are central issues. Loneliness may be the most powerful cause of affairs (Gottman and Gottman 2024). It may set the stage for the avalanche that follows.

Even though this chapter is primarily addressed to the IP, you, the HP, are also invited to consider the material and do the exercises. Some of the processes described may also be part of your experience.

# The Path To Betrayal

*Much of the material in this section is based on and adapted from the Gottman-Glass-Rusbult Hypothesized Cascade Toward Betrayal (Gottman and Gottman 2018).*

In the flow of relationship life, there are moments of deep connection as well as moments of disconnection. Your closeness ebbs and flows based on a multitude of issues: your job, your general state of mind, and other stressors you're facing. This means, at times, you will be exhausted, depleted, not at your best. You'll need things from your partner that they're not able to provide. Sometimes you may not even be aware of what you need from them. But often, there is some sense of loss or aloneness. Things just aren't as they should be.

This ebb and flow doesn't justify infidelity. It certainly didn't cause it. There was still choice involved and other options at every step along the way. It does, however, shine a light on aspects of your relationship that may have created distance and led to a pattern of avoidance. While the presence of these issues poses challenges, they're also a call to correction and connection.

The exercises in this chapter are for both of you. In the spirit of exploration and discovery, this chapter is designed to help both partners step back and analyze themes, patterns, and relationship dynamics that may have contributed to the betrayal. The conversations that will follow require use of all the communication skills you've developed. Remember, this is not a chapter to just *get past*, it's a process to *work through*. You both need to feel seen and heard. Your work in this chapter is part of the foundation of the new relationship you're creating.

Please complete each exercise individually, entering your responses in your journal.

After completing all of them, review your responses and make any additions or corrections that add clarity to your perspective.

Then, find a calm time to share what you wrote and discuss each section with your partner. It's generally a good idea to begin with a focus on the IP's position. This is the information the HP needs to understand.

It's usually wise to discuss this material in several shorter conversations rather than one marathon interaction.

Remember to be mindful, breathe, and take breaks when necessary. This is not material to rush through.

> ### Exercise: **Beginning the Exploration: How Did We Get Here?**
>
> As you begin this chapter, please take a few minutes to explore your view of why the affair happened. Describe what you believe led to the betrayal. List three things you believe led to the infidelity in your journal.

## Exploring the Relationship: Seeing the Dance

Drift happens! We all experience it. While it's sometimes a conscious strategy, it's more commonly an insidious, unplanned, and even unconscious move away from anticipated negativity. It's often a dull pain, a kind of aloneness that feels bad but is difficult to pin down. It hurts! It leaves you feeling dissatisfied, uncomfortable, taken for granted. Perhaps even unloved. Drift weakens your bond. Over time, it creates a tear in the fabric of your relationship. Unchecked, drift transforms lovers into roommates and partners into strangers.

What happens next is crucial. Do you face it or flee? Engage or distance yourself? Do you turn to your partner and begin a dialogue, or do you stay subterranean in your distress? Over time, if not addressed, drift has a pervasive, dampening impact on your experience of your relationship. It drains you of vitality, individually and collectively. By not sharing your feelings of disconnect or loneliness with your partner, you become even more distant. While it may avoid a negative, or even explosive exchange in the moment, you pay an incalculable cost over time. It leaves you alone in your pain.

This is not to say that you should just automatically blurt what you're feeling at any time of day or night. There are moments, times of emotional dysregulation, exhaustion, or a foul mood, when deferring the discussion to another time is prudent. The key issue here is that the engagement is merely being deferred to a better time. It is not being ignored.

Drift can be something experienced by both of you or it could be primarily an individual experience.

With your bond weakened, your pain elevated, and the perception "you're just not that into me" confirmed, the dance begins.

Do you see a pattern of drift in your relationship? Did you begin to feel less connected?

### Exercise: Detecting Drift

Think back to times when you noticed drift in your relationship. Use your journal to list two times when you drifted and two times when you felt your partner drifted.

#### Times When I Drifted

- How did I drift away from my partner? What did it look like?
- When I noticed it, how did I respond?
- Upon reflection, how do I wish I had handled it?

#### Times When My Partner Drifted

- How did my partner drift away from me? What did it look like?
- Did they notice it? How did they respond?
- How do you think they wish they had handled it?

## Turning Away

In the normal flow of everyday relationship life, you interact with your partner. You talk about your plans for the day. Who's taking the kids to school, to soccer practice, what do you think about dinner? You might share a concern or a joy. But in the atmosphere of drift, you do so less and less. This is a somewhat typical issue for partners sliding toward betrayal. As your turning away increases, even when your partner does reach for you, it doesn't register. You don't respond to it. As a result, you become even less engaged and less responsive to your partner. At some point, when they too pull back, you do notice that. You begin to feel you're the one doing all the work.

In this situation, you may more consciously turn away from your partner. You feel your partner has communicated that you're not important to them. So now you turn away, feeling a sense of justification. Once this sense of justification had taken root, there's an odd quality to your turning away. You believe it's your partner's fault. And as your partner experiences your lack of responsiveness, or even overt rejection, their energy to approach you fades. This becomes a self-perpetuating loop.

Reaching for even a moment of engagement with your partner requires initiative. Someone must take the risk of approaching. It's called a *bid for connection* (Gottman and Gottman 2024). There's some compelling relationship data about these seemingly small events. When partners are in a good place with each other, bids are received and responded to in a positive manner 86 percent of the time. When I reach for you, you receive it and reach back…a connecting moment. This is enough to create a positive momentum of continuing to reach and engage. *I feel important to you.* Contrast this to partners who are not in a good place with each other. In this situation, when I reach, you receive and respond positively only 33 percent of the time…67 percent of the time you turn away or turn against me. This quickly devolves into a "why bother?" mindset. When we believe that our efforts to connect are unwanted, we quickly learn to stop reaching.

This combination of drift and turning away has you leaning out. The trajectory is clearly toward disconnection.

Did you notice yourself turning away from your partner?

> ### Exercise: **Bids and Turning Away**
>
> This is an important exercise. It begins to shed light on those moments, large and small, that accelerated the pattern of disconnection. It's designed to help you notice those moments that either move you closer or further apart.
>
> Once again, use your journal.
>
> #### Times When My Partner Turned Away
>
> Describe a moment when you reached for your partner and they didn't engage. They turned away from or against you. They ignored you or were negative toward you.
>
> - Describe what your partner did or failed to do.
> - How did you feel? How did it impact you?
> - What did you do?
>
> #### Times When I Turned Away
>
> Describe a time when your partner reached for you and you didn't engage. You turned away from or against them. You ignored them or were negative toward them.
>
> - Describe what you did or failed to do.
> - How did you explain or justify your behavior to yourself?
> - How do you think your partner felt? How did it impact them?
> - What did they do?

# The Impact of Vulnerability

The belief that your partner has turned away from you creates a sense of vulnerability. It's an uncomfortable state to be in. It can't be endured indefinitely. You may seek a way out. One way to escape that sense of vulnerability is to entertain the possibility of finding somebody else. A new person, a fresh start. Someone who sees your goodness and values you for who you are as a person. Just the idea of finding that new person may calm you.

## Negative Comparisons

The brilliant work of Caryl Rusbult explains what happens next. Her Investment Model of Commitment identified *negative comparisons* as a turning point (Rusbult, Martz, and Agnew 1998). As you, the IP, drift and turn away, something even more pernicious begins to bubble inside. You begin to make negative comparisons between your partner and "others." That "other" might be an actual person, perhaps someone at the office, at the coffeeshop, or at church. It could be a fantasized "other," like the movie star who would be just right for you, or a "hypothetical other," the "someone out there" who must be better for you. Someone who you're imagining would be nicer to you, perhaps more attentive, maybe even someone who would find you attractive or could make you happier than your partner. Someone who would appreciate you for who you are. And once these negative comparisons take root, you naturally gather data or notice moments that support them. You create a file that dramatically colors your perception of your partner.

You shift from valuing and cherishing the partner you have to demeaning and trashing them. First in your head, later in conversations with others. This negative redefining of your partner and your relationship has disastrous consequences as it deepens.

---

### Exercise: **Negative Comparisons**

Identify a moment when you made a negative comparison regarding your partner. Write it in your journal.

- What was the message you gave yourself?
- What did you feel?

- Did you combat it with a positive thought about your partner or give it room to grow?
- Did you share it with your partner?
- Do you believe your partner has made negative comparisons about you?
- What do you think they felt?
- Do you think they countered it with a positive thought of you or gave it room to grow?

## Dark Glasses: A Negative Lens

In this situation, when you do address an issue, it goes badly. You enter with a negative point of view—with dark-colored glasses. You're in a state called *negative sentiment override* (Gottman and Gottman 2024). Let's just call it a *negative perspective:* a term for an atmosphere where negativity thrives and positivity withers. You're wearing dark glasses that affect all you see.

In this negative perspective, you automatically scan for negativity. A destructive corollary is that you're also less likely to notice the positives expressed by your partner (Robinson and Price 1980). Their kind words and thoughtful actions don't register. It's as if they didn't offer them. You systematically minimize the positivity of your partner. You fail to give the benefit of the doubt. You perceive, emphasize, and nurture the negatives you've gathered about them. You're likely to experience your partner's words and actions more negatively than they intended. In this darkened, distorted world, conflict escalates quickly. You're trapped in a *negative absorbing state* (Gottman and Gottman 2018). You don't see a solution. Nothing you do to try to change it works.

Part of the problem is that you may perceive your partner as being the source of the negativity in conversations. In that state, you feel like the aggrieved party and it's your partner's responsibility to be nicer, more polite, more positive. You're waiting for them to lighten up. You might even begin to shift the fundamental way you view your partner. Rather than cherishing them, as you once did, you begin to trash them. First in your head and perhaps later while talking with others. You no longer see them as the kind, interesting person you fell in love with. They no longer feel like your future. They now are seen as an adversary.

This negative perspective is crucial to understanding the escalating distance and disconnect that follows. Once this negative perspective has taken root, it feels like nothing works. Even positive words, with positive intent, fall on deaf ears.

### Exercise: **The Atmosphere Darkens**

Describe a situation when you could only see your partner through a negative lens. When whatever they said or did affected you in the wrong way.

- What did you notice?
- How did it impact you?
- What did you do?

When you think of it now, can you think of a way you could offer some grace to your partner? A way you could give them the benefit of the doubt?

Describe a situation when you believe your partner could only see you through a negative lens. When your words and actions were interpreted as negative, even though that was not your intent.

- What do you think they noticed?
- How do you think these words and actions impacted them?
- What did they do?
- How do you wish they would have responded?

## Resentment

Resentment contaminates! It's here that you deepen the shift from cherishing your partner to trashing them. With pain as your guide and your perception of your partner jaded, you no longer see them as the kind, caring, loving person you fell in love with. You see them as self-centered.

The word you may use to describe their essence is "selfish"! As you struggle with feeling lonely and seeing no way back from the edge, hope fades.

---

**Exercise: Resentment Rules**

Describe how resentment entered your relationship:

- What led you to change how you viewed your partner?
- Was there a particular moment, a specific event?
- What did you begin to tell yourself about them?
- As that narrative deepened, did you challenge it or simply go with it?
- Over time, how did it impact how you treated your partner?

---

## Flooding and the Four Horsemen

By this point in the process, with the negative perspective in ascendance, it's common for both of you to be susceptible to two communication killers: flooding and the Four Horsemen. If you and your partner tend to avoid conflict, you may not experience these destructive communication patterns very often. Or when they do surface, they will be brief and transient. If however, you're inclined to address issues, they more frequently come to the forefront. When you discuss a topic in the negative perspective, it goes poorly. In fact, it's common for a topic to morph into an "issue," then quickly become a "problem" based on the way you interact with each other.

When you begin to butt heads with your partner and it feels like an adversarial exchange, your nervous system senses danger or threat. In those moments your body reacts, preparing to protect you. This physiological activation is called *flooding* (Gottman and Gottman 2018). It's more commonly referred to as "fight or flight." It should be noted that fight or flight is not necessarily a pathological or dysfunctional state. It's a deeply embedded instinct that serves you well in situations of perceived danger or threat. It's essential to your survival. The relational implications, however, are important to be mindful of. In fight or flight, you operate from an individual rather than a relational perspective. You shift to a survival focus, not a relationship focus.

When engaged in distressing conflict with your partner, your body is triggered. Your heart quickens, you secrete stress hormones. A cascade of physiological changes prepares you for battle. In intimate relationships, it's not unusual to secrete a combination of adrenaline and cortisol. Adrenaline is an activating stress hormone…it moves you to "do" something. "Don't just sit there…take action." You might raise your voice, pound on the table, or get in your partner's face. Cortisol, on the other hand, is a stress hormone that promotes "passive coping." It leaves you feeling powerless. You tend to feel hopeless. You might shut down, possibly to try to disengage. You might be moved to leave the room. In these moments, healthy communication is unlikely.

This physiological activation is intense and depleting. In your desperation to deal with the perceived threat coming from your partner, you move to a sort of automatic pilot. Your physiology and emotions guide your words and actions. Your ability to take in your partner's words and hear them accurately is compromised.

When flooded, you're hypersensitive to slights and put-downs. You experience your partner as being negative. A destructive communication pattern opens. The Four Horsemen, criticism, defensiveness, contempt, and stonewalling enter (Gottman and Gottman 2024). Negative emotions escalate, hurts accelerate, and the tendency to be reactive is triggered. You may say some of your ugliest things during moments of flooding. A cycle of criticism and defensiveness opens. Contempt and stonewalling may follow.

# The Path to Infidelity

The negative impacts of flooding and the Four Horsemen are pernicious. They can become pervasive. You don't see a way out of the negative escalation. Repair efforts rarely work (Gottman and Gottman 2024). Nothing works.

At this point, you're inaccessible. You don't accept influence. When your partner speaks, you don't take it in as your rebuttal brain takes over (Gottman and Gottman 2024). You settle behind a wall of self-righteousness. Another brick has been added to the wall. Your view of your partner becomes a negative absorbing state. The central characteristic of a negative absorbing state is that, while it's easy to enter, it's difficult to escape. You find fault with everything they say or do. You invest less in the relationship.

> **Exercise: Identify Your Communication Issues**
>
> *Flooding.* Can you tell when you move into *fight or flight?*
>
> > What do you notice in your body? Heart palpitations, neck tension, a queasy stomach, or a dry mouth? These are but a few of many possible bodily sensations you might experience.
> >
> > Do you notice how difficult it is to really listen to your partner? Not only do you need to talk, but you receive their words with a pervasive negative spin.
> >
> > How do you calm yourself and reset your nervous system?
> >
> > Do you know how to take a break and then return to the conversation?
>
> *Four Horsemen.* Can you think of a time when your tone and words became negative and attacking?
>
> > When you moved into criticism or contempt, looking and talking down to your partner?
> >
> > When your reaction was to defend yourself and explain or justify your position?

> Or when you began to shut down or withdraw? When you wanted to escape?
>
> *Repair.* Repair is an essential process to recover from damaging, distancing moments. Without it, wounds fester and hurts deepen. During a fight or after the conflict, did you try to get back on track and repair the conversation?
>
> *Accept Influence.* In moments of upset, could you step out of your own position and see even a bit of truth in your partner's position, even if you disagree with it? Could you sense their pain? Did you have any compassion for them?
>
> Bottom line: flooding and the Four Horsemen make the idea of even trying to talk feel like a losing proposition. Why bother? It's just going to deteriorate.

# The Pivot to Avoidance

So now, having drifted apart and turned away, you feel alone. With negative comparisons taking root and an atmosphere colored by negative sentiment override, you feel discouraged. Your efforts to communicate are blocked by flooding, the Four Horsemen, failed repair, and an inability to accept influence. In these circumstances, avoidance seems like a reasonable idea. And in a way, it is reasonable…or at least understandable. And in the big picture, over the course of a time, it's a disastrous path to take. *Avoidance kills!*

When avoidance becomes the default setting, you make fewer bids for connection, engage less, and share less with your partner. You may even choose to not share the mundane, basic events of your day with your partner. You certainly don't risk sharing your deeper feelings or bringing up areas of upset or dissatisfaction. And you do this with a sense of justification. The justification that your partner is impossible. That you've tried, you've made real efforts, that you've reached out…all to no avail. When is enough *enough*? Why do you continue to put yourself through this? This litany of self-justifying self-talk closes the case.

# The Path to Infidelity

In *Not Just Friends* (2003), Shirley Glass described two types of avoidance that are particularly problematic. One is *conflict avoidance,* the systematic moving away from topics or moments of tension with your partner. This has a negative impact on your relationship because it eliminates the natural process of addressing issues that are causing upset or distress. There's no path to healing hurts or treating wounds. In this context, they grow and deepen in the dark.

The second destructive type of avoidance is *self-disclosure avoidance.* This pattern of not bringing your thoughts, feelings, wants, wishes, and needs to your partner leaves them in the dark and you feeling alone. Of course you have reasons for taking this path. You may feel your partner wouldn't be receptive or even care about your concerns. And there may even be some truth to your feelings. But the problem is that, when this becomes the norm, the bridge between you is closed.

The irony is that even as you, the IP, move away from your partner and avoid interacting with them, you're internally convinced that it's their fault. So, the gap widens, the rut deepens, and what was once a crack now becomes a chasm.

This is an important element in the slide to betrayal. Once you arrive at this juncture, there's likely no possibility of resolving issues or healing hurts.

---

### Exercise: **The Decision to Avoid**

Think of times when you turned to avoidance rather than addressing issues or feelings. Describe the shift in your journal. As you became more avoidant, what did you notice? What did you feel?

Describe a situation when you opted to avoid a conflict rather than risk addressing it:

- How did it feel?
- What were the benefits?
- What were the costs?

Now, describe a moment when you decided to avoid self-disclosure: when you took the path of keeping an important feeling or need to yourself, rather than sharing it with your partner:

- How did it feel?

- What was the benefit?

- What was the cost?

Now, as you look back on the pattern of avoidance, what story or narrative led you to take that path? Describe what you were telling yourself about your partner, or their likely reaction if you did bring the issue to them.

- When you look back, how did that decision impact your relationship?

- What were the benefits?

- What were the costs?

Now, perhaps most importantly, what do you wish you had done differently? Describe what you'll do differently in the future.

## Secrets

You've now laid the groundwork for keeping secrets. You see your partner as the problem. Secrecy begins with avoidance behaviors. You may stop telling your partner the details of your day, small events that describe your daily life. It eventually includes anything you believe might create conflict. *Why bother? Nothing good will come of it.* With avoidance firmly entrenched, it becomes a way of life.

At this point, you move beyond simply avoiding conflict and avoiding self-disclosure to omitting information, thoughts, feelings, or experiences that you know have a direct impact on your relationship. Moments of doubt about your future together, feelings of excitement or attraction when talking with a co-worker, and perhaps even visualizing what life with another partner might be like.

It may also include actual moments spent with that coworker. Long coffee breaks, "business" lunches, "supportive" conversations about their relationship struggles. While in real time you may have felt those interactions were innocent, collegial or just friendly, this is the time for you to take a deeper look. Upon reflection, these are clearly things your partner needed to know about.

When you notice doubts regarding the viability of your relationship or an increasing attraction or excitement about interactions with another person, it's time to talk. These are not easy things to talk about. They're uncomfortable to face. Yet, not doing so permits them to take root and grow.

---

### Exercise: **Secrets Separate Us**

With the idea of secrets open in your consciousness, revisit those negative relationship thoughts and negative comparisons you made about your partner. Re-examine those "innocent" interactions with others.

Describe any negative thoughts you began to have about your partner and your relationship. Not just something that popped up once and vanished, but those things that became recurrent.

Now, use your journal to describe any interactions with another person that you now realize were more than innocent, collegial or friendly. While they may not have been overtly flirtatious or sexualized, you knew you were near or over the line. They were too personal, intimate, or exciting. You looked forward to them too much.

What kept you from bringing this to your partner?

What do you wish you had discussed with your partner?

---

## Crossing the Line

Now, with the slide into keeping secrets in full swing, you're at risk of crossing the line into infidelity. It's possible you've already moved into the territory of an emotional affair.

Imagine that you see someone in the coffeeshop line who smiles at you. You notice and strike up a bit of conversation. Just being friendly, nothing wrong with this. But you head for the same coffeeshop again the next morning, eyes expectant, hoping they'll be there too. You make a point of engaging. They smile again. They're friendly. The slippery slope calls.

The pivotal factor here is that you notice a feeling and fail to take heed or talk with your partner about it. *Of course you don't need to. It wasn't that big of a deal, just a social hello to a stranger,* you tell yourself. But if you're honest, it was a bit more than that. You were looking forward to it. You hoped they would be there. Another secret, but this time it was easy.

In the book *Not Just Friends,* Shirley Glass calls this a shift of "walls and windows." As the wall rises between you and your partner, a window opens with your newfound friend. Over time, one thing leads to another. The path from the coffeeshop to their apartment happened so naturally.

---

### Exercise: How It "Just Happened"

This is a challenging exercise to describe in your journal. Here you're asked to break free of the justification that enabled you to cross the line. You're asked to see and own the decision you made.

Describe the time you brought the "windows and walls" dynamic into your relationship. When you moved away from your partner and toward another person. This is different than just having a friend. It's about actively choosing another person over your partner. In a sense, it's done at your partner's expense. As painful as it might be…tell the story in your journal.

---

Let's now spend a few moments looking at loneliness and vulnerability. These issues are important as you continue to move forward.

### *Loneliness*

Loneliness is a crucial topic for both of you to explore. For you, the Involved Partner, it may be a central part of the slide into betrayal. Part of how you justified the path you walked. It may also be something you experience or fear now as you look to the future, unsure of what lies ahead.

For you, the Hurt Partner, loneliness is a complicated experience. Your world has been turned upside down. The past may seem like a lie, the present is pain and the future is uncertain. As you grapple with the betrayal, loneliness intensifies and concerns about the future deepen.

When you're lonely over an extended period of time, your level of happiness plummets and your internal degree of negativity rises. Chronic loneliness is also bad for you physically. It compromises your immune system (Cacioppo 1990). And the loneliness you're now experiencing, loneliness while in a relationship, is especially devastating

Take a few minutes to complete this exercise on loneliness. It's important for you to recognize and let your partner in on your loneliness.

---

### Exercise: My Loneliness

Open your journal and describe your experience of loneliness in this relationship.

- Describe what you felt then and how you feel now.
- How did you cope with it?
- How do you wish you had responded to it?
- What did you need from your partner?

---

### *Vulnerability*

Vulnerability is an unavoidable aspect of intimate relationships. It's part of being known. You can't feel close without it. And yet, as essential as it is, you likely naturally move away from it. Especially now, in the wake of betrayal. It's uncomfortable. It leaves you at risk. The self-protective voice within says, *If I let you in, you could hurt me again, and that hurt is more than I can endure.* So, you move away.

Vulnerability can be destabilizing. Accepting vulnerability, opening your heart to your partner, is difficult. Becoming comfortable with it is the work of a lifetime. It's also the work you'll face in the next chapter.

---

**Exercise: The Value of Vulnerability**

Recall a time when you took the risk to be vulnerable with your partner.

- What did you share with them?
- What led you to take that risk? How did you decide to let them in?
- How did your partner respond?
- Would you do it again?

---

# In Closing

This was a difficult chapter. Slowing down and really examining betrayal is painful work. While not all of these situations are part of your story, it's likely that some are. This work offers clarity about some of the issues you need to face. As you understand what happened, your confusion will begin to clear. You'll gain some insight about yourself, your partner, and your relationship. This will serve as a guide as you rebuild your relationship.

CHAPTER 10

# Attachment: Commitment and Intimacy

There was a time, without knowing what the future held, when you chose one another. You committed to one another, forsaking all others. Did you know what you were signing up for? Perhaps not. Neither of you knew what life would bring. But one thing you did know: you knew *who* you were choosing to travel with.

Alain Badiou, a French philosopher, speaks of love being a chance encounter, and depending on the path you create and how you walk that path, love has the potential to feel like destiny (Badiou 2009). This is your second chance to make a first impression and create that path.

Caryl Rusbult's Investment Model of Commitment helps us understand that commitment can be nurtured and developed; it's not just something you either have or you don't (Rusbult, Agnew, and Arriaga 2011). The more you invest in your relationship, the stronger your commitment. And the deeper your level of commitment, the more you'll invest. In this sense, you chose commitment rather than just waiting for it to happen. So if commitment is your choice, how do you do it? Simple, you invest and engage. In difficult moments, you turn toward and engage rather than opting to withdraw or avoid. You permit the things you love about your partner and your relationship to quiet the frustration of the moment and do the work of building your bond. You now have the skills to do this in a balanced, loving, respectful way. Knowing the dangers associated with avoidance, leaning in is the only option.

## Considering Commitment

Where do you stand today on the issue of commitment? Can you commit to a future together? Are you ready to commit to a future together?

Commitment is an active process, not a passive one. It's the idea that "I choose you today and every day. In my words, actions, and priorities."

Emotional and physical intimacy are at the heart of this chapter. You'll be asked to share things closer to the heart. You'll be invited to begin to "dream" again. What do you want, what do you need?

Can you take the risk of being vulnerable and truly letting your partner in? In the wake of betrayal, this can feel risky…and it is. Moving beyond being able to live together to being able to love together involves an openness that leaves you vulnerable. Do the skills you've developed and the trust you now feel give you the courage for yet another leap of faith?

The trust you now have in yourself is also part of the commitment decision. The knowledge that no matter what happens, you'll be okay, is crucial. It impacts your comfort with sharing, risking, and reaching for each other in the relationship.

Commitment also encompasses the deeper themes of life dreams and life meaning or purpose. Your time on this planet is finite: it will come to an end someday. How do you choose to spend the time gifted to you? Who do you want to spend it with?

# Deepening Friendship

Let's begin with an old-fashioned word that may have found new meaning in the way you think of your partner: *cherishing*. It's an essential aspect of commitment. It's an antidote to resentment. Cherishing is a natural defense against the cascade toward betrayal. When I cherish you, I'm taken by the things I love and value about you. They outweigh the frustrations of the moment. Despite moments of tension, you remain the person I chose at the beginning and choose again today and every day. It implies a deep knowing, appreciation, and valuing of who you are and what you bring to the relationship. There's a recognition of the person *I* become in your presence. Being with you makes me a better person. Cherishing is part of commitment. Cherishing conveys the feeling that I see you as unique and irreplaceable.

## Solving the Moment

As you focus on deeper levels of connection, the idea of "solving the moment" jumps to the head of the class. It invites you to step out of self-importance and be truly mindful of and present with your partner. It's less about being sacrificial and more about giving grace. This type of emotional intimacy is particularly critical in moments when your partner is struggling. When they're hurting, it's your opportunity to be there for them. Tune into their hurt and move toward them. Don't leave them alone in their pain.

Another aspect of emotional intimacy is about you being more open and vulnerable. It requires stepping out of your image of yourself to let your partner see the real you. Becoming a bit more comfortable with being vulnerable is a skill worth developing. Perhaps you never get fully "comfortable" with vulnerability, but it's a skill you can develop.

## Life Dreams and Shared Meaning

As you work to increase your level of attachment and create more emotional intimacy in your relationship, life dreams and shared meaning come to the forefront of your mind.

### *Life Dreams*

Dreams reside deep within the human psyche. They live in you too. Take some time to revisit the history of your dreams. What were your life dreams before you met your partner? What happened to them after you met? Were those dreams built into the life you created with your partner? Did you honor them or perhaps give up on them?

Do you feel entitled to dream? What are your life dreams, those things in life that carry great meaning to you, now? Is your partner aware of your dreams? Do you know theirs? How does your partner show that they care about your dreams? How do you send that message to them? Do they actively support your dreams?

The trauma of betrayal is life disruptive. It isn't conducive to dreaming. No matter what your intellect says, you may not feel free to dream.

## Exercise: Dream a Little Dream

Use your journal to work on describing and honoring your life dreams.

- What were your most important life dreams before you met your partner?
- After becoming a couple, what were your most important *individual* life dreams?
- How are those dreams part of your life today? Describe how you live them. What do they contribute to your overall life satisfaction?
- If they're not part of your life today, describe the cost you pay. What are you missing out on and how does that impact you?
- Describe one individual dream that would make a real difference to you today if you found a way to add it to your life experience.
- What can you do to make that dream come true?

Think back to a time early in your relationship.

- What were your dreams for the relationship?
- How are those dreams part of your life today? Describe how you live them. What do they contribute to your overall life satisfaction?
- If they're not part of your life today, describe the cost you pay. What are you missing out on and how does that impact you?
- Describe one relationship dream that would make a real difference to you today if you found a way to add it to your life experience.
- What can you do to make that dream come true?

# Shared Meaning and Life Purpose

As human beings, we're fated to try to make sense out of the time we have on this planet. At this level, we're all philosophers. What is our existence about? Why are we here? What's the point of being on this fragile, spinning globe? In *Man's Search for Meaning*, Viktor Frankl reflects on his experience as a prisoner in Nazi concentration camps and sheds some light on the elusive topic of humanity and life meaning: He suggests that the path to meaning involves something beyond self-interest, that the pursuit of individual happiness is not the goal. Life meaning is connected to making a difference in the world, to making a contribution to others.

In the wake of betrayal, it's important to revisit your values. Discuss what you identify as your guiding principles as you move forward. Commit to the ethical and moral positions embedded in those principles. They may also be reflected in your spiritual and religious beliefs and practices. This category calls you to your higher self. Your values are revealed in your words and actions. By where you spend your time, energy and resources.

Start by exploring the importance of creating shared meaning with your partner. What do you need to feel that the life you share has purpose?

You came from different families, with different ways of living. You grew up witnessing the benefits and shortcomings of the culture you were born into. As you and your partner came together, you too created a culture. Your own way of living that emphasized some ideas, behaviors, and values while disregarding others. Perhaps it centered around your personal bond and the joy of time together. You might have come together with the focus on raising kids and having a family, creating wealth, helping others, or becoming part of a larger community.

Wherever you started, it's fair to say that the beginning focus has likely evolved and changed, at least a bit, over time. Life presents unexpected opportunities and challenges. A dream job that requires a geographic relocation, the loss of a family member, twins rather than one bundle of joy, a miscarriage, cancer, a "sure thing" investment that goes bad. These unplanned, unanticipated events affected you. They changed you. They changed your relationship. When these life-altering events entered your life, you made another important decision…did you face them together?

You're at another life juncture. The opportunity and challenge to explore and share the things that lend meaning to your time on this planet. The moral, ethical, and perhaps spiritual principles at the center of the life you created have been violated by the betrayal. It's time to revisit and update those values. To look again at what you need and what you're willing to endeavor to create. This is an opportunity for you as individuals, as well as for you as partners.

A sense of shared meaning doesn't just happen. You need to be intentional. This means deciding how you will move through time together (Gottman and Gottman 2024).

Here are three categories to consider:

1. Start by creating *rituals of connection*. These rituals provide a basic flow to life. Create rituals to celebrate formal occasions like your anniversary, birthdays, or holidays. Also create rituals around daily living: sharing meals together, exercising, finding time to talk, and making time for physical intimacy.

2. Discuss *shared life goals* and the mission you both feel compelled to achieve. These are aspirational ideas that motivate you.

3. Be mindful of the *multiple roles* you each fill…partner, parent, friend…and have conversations about the kind of support that would be meaningful to you in each area.

The Life Dreams and Shared Meaning exercises are meant to start as journal work for each of you; then share and discuss them together.

## Exercise: Informal Rituals: Daily Living

*Create daily or weekly rituals of connection.* Rituals offer dependable patterns of connection. An essential element of impactful, sustainable rituals is that they have personal meaning for both of you. Remember, the spirit under each ritual is about being emotionally present and creating a moment of connection. In this mindset, even small moments can yield big results. Add these to your journal. Then discuss them with your partner.

1. *Waking Ritual.* Start your day in a way that sets a positive tone for the day. When you open your eyes in the morning, what would feel good to you? A welcoming word, warm hug, or hot cup of coffee? Do you share a few words before picking up your phone, or is your phone the vehicle for connection? Come up with a ritual you'll both feel good about and try it for a week. Make adjustments as necessary.

2. Describe the morning ritual in your journal.

3. *Together Again Ritual.* How do you mark the transition from the workday to your personal life? The first ten minutes matter. While every couple's life flow is different, the key here is to come up with something that leaves both of you feeling seen, heard and cared about. It sets the tone for the rest of the evening. It might be a twenty-second hug the moment you lay eyes on each other. It could take the form of a mini-emotional check-in. "How are you feeling? What's on your mind? What do you need right now?" Leading with "I'm glad you're home. I missed you. It's really nice to see you" is a nice opening touch. Sharing how you're feeling and what you hope for during the evening is of value too.

4. Describe the together again ritual in your journal.

5. *Bedtime Ritual.* This end-of-the-day ritual carries the benefit of a peaceful, personal connection before sleep. It may include snuggling and affection...or perhaps not. Touch is a

complicated topic following betrayal. Describe what would feel welcome and reassuring to you now.

6. Describe the bedtime ritual in your journal.

There are a multitude of additional rituals you might consider. For instance, date nights, cooking together, sharing mealtimes, the flow of the evening, nature walks, exercise, adventure, and time with close friends are all worth discussion. After working on rituals in your journal, set a time to discuss these informal rituals with your partner.

A key to creating successful rituals is to approach them with enough specificity that both of you have clarity about the logistics and expectations. Be clear about who will initiate the ritual, what each partner will do, how it will start and end, and how often you will do each ritual. Being clear is a good beginning.

Remember, these rituals are designed to create patterns of connection and to serve you. They're not meant to be legalistic contracts that then become the source of conflict or dispute. Exceptions happen. Approach them with grace. And if you decide a particular ritual isn't working for you, set a time to talk.

## Exercise: Formal Rituals—Life Events

Before beginning this exercise, it's helpful to revisit your life experience with special events. You carry a mental "file" within that is the context from which your rituals arise. You may be moved to recapture something from your past. On the other hand, you may be committed to creating something different. Start with your childhood, then adolescence and adulthood. How did your family celebrate special days…or not? How did they impact you? What did they mean to you?

Special events have the potential to live inside you long after the day has passed. Take the time to review your history. What did special events mean to you then? What do they mean to you now? Share the stories of your past, as well as your hopes for the future.

*Anniversary.* This ritual is about more than remembering the date of your wedding or commitment ceremony. It's about reexperiencing being chosen. Do you still feel chosen? It's about your sense of gratitude for having the privilege of spending yet another year together.

*Birthday.* Here the theme is also more than a reminder in your phone that your partner was born on this date. It's a marker of another year in your partner's time on this planet and another year together. It's an opportunity to look back as well as look forward, and honor the birthday person.

*Holiday or Religious Celebration.* There are many events to choose from here. Select one that has particular significance to you. Revisit how you experienced it as a younger person. What it meant to you. Now create a day around that holiday this year. Be as detailed as you can about the flow of the day, weekend, or week. Not all events are limited to a single day. Agree on the logistics of who will do what, when, where, and how. Being clear is a good beginning.

Discuss the kind of rituals that would be most meaningful to you.

## Exercise: Individual and Relationship Goals

As life unfolds, your days tend to fill with responsibilities, duties and activities. Circumstances change. Raising kids, caring for aging parents, and participating in community can all demand time and attention. Careers change. Your personal health changes. These *normal* life experiences place limits on your time, resources, and energy. As you're swept along by the tide of life, it's crucial to take the time to consciously, intentionally prioritize the things you value the most (Doherty 1997). This is particularly salient in the wake of betrayal.

The goals you set together will go a long way in determining the path you create and walk together. What goals do you have for yourself? For your relationship? Consider the following questions:

- What goals do you have for this year? For 5 years from now?
- What goals feel compelling?
- What do you need to add or subtract to have more balance in your life?
- What do you aspire to?
- How do you want to be remembered?

Work on your goals in your journal, then discuss these goals with your partner.

> ## Exercise: Roles
>
> Life roles tend to increase over time. The roles you emphasize define your path. Be mindful of where you dedicate your time and resources. No one, not even you, can be everything to everyone. Perhaps you've tried this before. Make these choices with your values and core needs in mind.
>
> Here are some roles that might be part of your life: partner, parent, grandparent, son, daughter, sibling, friend, employee, boss, neighbor, or community member. Let me suggest you add one more that's frequently overlooked…yourself. Be conscious of the importance of developing and nurturing a relationship with yourself.
>
> Now, go to your journal and prioritize these roles. Determine which are essential and must be part of your life and which are optional.
>
> Make another entry describing the participation or support you would like from your partner. Then discuss them with your partner.

# Sexual Intimacy

*The exercises in this section are for both of you to work on individually and then to discuss together when it feels right. This is not a conversation to force or feel forced into.*

Physical intimacy is such a personal issue. Such a difficult issue in the wake of infidelity. The most personal expression of intimacy between you and your partner has been contaminated by another person. Even if you've made the decision to try to bring a physical connection back into your relationship, it's complicated. The trauma of infidelity and the related emotional upheaval make any simple approach to physical intimacy elusive. There's a clear link between close, personal, connecting touch, affection, sex, and emotional intimacy. The more secure you feel, the more comfortable you are with being vulnerable. The more trust has been built and commitment reestablished, the safer sex feels.

You may desire to return to something you once experienced together or to how it was prior to the betrayal. Or you may want it to be different.

You may be drawn to touch or you may avoid it—maybe both. You may feel violated at the thought or perhaps reassured. What feels right to you in one moment can change in a flash. This is the nature of trauma. Touch can feel warm and comforting only to be suddenly contaminated by the intrusive thought of your partner doing the same thing with their affair partner. The terrain is tenuous. Are you ready to talk about physical intimacy? What you want or don't want, like or don't like; what you're ready for; or perhaps more importantly, what you're not ready for. And no matter how you feel today, you might feel differently tomorrow. The trauma of betrayal makes this a crucial issue. Your feelings and readiness must be the guide. (Gottman and Gottman 2024).

## Where to Begin

While there aren't universal rules to follow when it comes to physical intimacy following infidelity, here's an idea to begin with: *don't force it*. Don't push yourself to engage in behaviors that don't feel right to you. Don't put yourself in positions that will only cause more anguish or self-doubt. An intimate physical relationship begins with being true to yourself. Honor yourself and how you feel in the moment.

### *Sex Begins Before the Bedroom*

Emotional intimacy is the foundation from which sexual intimacy emerges. In long-term, committed relationships, sex is part of a larger, deeper connection. That connection is formed in the fabric of your daily living together. As you move through the day, you notice, turn toward, and lean in toward one another. You know your partner and feel known by them. You value them and feel valued by them. These are the conditions of emotional intimacy. In this bubble, as you interact, you might flirt, touch, or include sexual innuendo in your comments. In this regard, you might say that "everything is sex." All you do and say throughout the day, as it connects you, is a form of foreplay. When you feel close, seen, heard, and safe with your partner, the conditions for sex begin to bubble.

A groundbreaking book *The Normal Bar* reported data from an international study reaching 70,000 people in twenty-four countries (Northrup,

Schwartz, and Witte 2013). They addressed the issue of what differentiates people who say they have a great sex life from those who don't. They discovered that couples around the globe, with thriving, satisfying sexual relationships, practiced similar habits. Here are some of those habits. Saying "I love you," kissing, and cuddling were part of their regular routine. They were physically affectionate and emotionally connected. They made romantic gestures and created romantic time together. They could talk about sex, knew their partner's sexual preferences, and built time for sex into their lives. Nothing too shocking, unusual, or kinky here. In fact, most of these things happened outside of the bedroom.

These findings emphasize the importance of emotional intimacy, friendship, and touch in couples who report a satisfying sexual relationship. And to be clear, the touch referenced here is not just sexual touch. Warm or affectionate touch is essential to your well-being. Without it, we struggle. *Touch deprivation* is linked to emotional distress (Field 2001).

## Nonsexual Touch

Nonsexual touch is an important component of sexual intimacy. The significance of touch is evidenced in a wide array of human relationships. Infants need the touch of their mothers to feel secure. Mothers need it too. Skin contact between moms and babies is life-giving to both of them. Nonsexual intimate physical touch triggers the release of oxytocin, a hormone that facilitates bonding and connection (Field 2001). Touch contributes to your physical health and longevity. When it comes to romantic relationships, couples who cuddle more have more satisfying long-term relationships. In *The Normal Bar*, only 6 percent of non-cuddling partners reported having a great sex life. It's clear that affectionate touch is connected to a thriving sex life (Gottman and Gottman 2022).

After the trauma of betrayal, the importance of nonsexual, affectionate touch may be even greater. This kind of touch carries a real sense of giving, not just receiving. It clearly conveys the message "you matter to me." While talking about sexual touch is awkward for many, talking about nonsexual, affectionate touch is more comfortable. This is the perfect opportunity to put words to your experience of touch as well as your preferences.

## Exercise: Talking About Nonsexual Touch

Think about your life history of being touched. Remember what it felt like as a child. Did a hug from Mom feel comforting but less so with Dad? Or was it the other way around? Did it feel different during adolescence, with your emerging sexuality beginning to bubble? What about physical embraces with friends or those close to you as a young adult? Was touch comfortable or did it leave you feeling uneasy?

Your "touch history" remains embedded in your nervous system even to this day. Some touch feels comfortable, other types less so.

Revisit your experience with nonsexual touch through the following questions. Describe what felt good and what didn't. Use your journal.

- What types of touch were most comforting to you? Give an example.
- What kinds of touch just never felt right? Give an example.
- When stressed, do you long for touch or do you find it even more distressing?
- Are there moments when you really need touch or a hug?
- Are there other times when that same touch would feel intrusive?

Now focus on your nonsexual touch history with your partner.

- What types of touch with your partner were most comforting to you? Give an example.
- What kinds of touch with your partner just never felt right? Give an example.
- When stressed, do you turn to your partner for touch, or turn away? Why?
- When you and your partner are touching, do you feel you're receiving or giving?

# Speaking of Sex

Emotional intimacy is the basis of your path to sexual intimacy. Before dealing with your partner's sexual wants, needs, and preferences, it's useful to take some time to explore what sexual intimacy means to you and what it looks like. In her insightful 2015 book *Come As You Are,* Emily Nagoski talks about the dual process model of sex. Here, she approaches sexuality from the perspective of getting to know yourself and understanding the origins of your "natural" sexual preferences: things you're comfortable with and drawn toward as well as those you're not comfortable with and tend to move away from. She refers to them as your sexual "brakes" and sexual "accelerators." It's important to note that your specific brakes and accelerators are a result of your lived experience. Your family background, culture, religious upbringing, society, and personal sexual experiences affect your views of sexuality. It's also crucial to understand that your unique brakes and accelerators make sense. Given the life you've lived, it's easy to see how they emerged. They're nothing to be ashamed of. They are something to be understood. As you recover from the trauma of infidelity, this is important work.

---

### Exercise: **Exploring Your Brakes and Accelerators**

Review your life story and the primary lessons you learned about sexuality. How did your own experiences add to the story? How does the infidelity impact it now? Use your journal.

- What conditions move you away from sex?
- What conditions move you toward sex?
- How has this betrayal impacted your "brake"?
- How has this betrayal impacted your "accelerator"?

> ### Exercise: **Where to Begin?**
>
> Take some time to explore how you feel about sexual intimacy. You may be comfortable with sexual touch or sexual activity or perhaps not. It may be too early. Perhaps certain types of sexual intimacy seem right, but not others. And even if you're already sexually active with your partner, take time to reconsider if it's right for you. This is an opportunity to reset the situation. Use your journal.
>
> - What am I comfortable with and ready for?
> - What feels uncomfortable and needs to be deferred until later?

## Creating the Conditions for Sexual Intimacy

As you create and walk the path to healthy sexual intimacy, you need to feel safe and comfortable with the direction and pace of your journey. This calls for calm, compassionate conversation. The following exercises create vulnerability. Be sure you're ready to talk before beginning. If it feels awkward or becomes too tense, take a break. This isn't the kind of material to force.

> ### Exercise: **Share Your Brakes and Accelerators**
>
> Review your journal entry about your brakes and accelerators. Share the parts you're ready to reveal. Hold off on the parts you're uncomfortable sharing. There will be other opportunities.

Part of saying "yes" to sex is being free to say "no." So, if you opt to say, "No, I'm just too tired or have too much on my mind," how does your partner respond? Do they get mad and berate you? Do they get pouty and abandon you? Do they become controlling and try to pressure you into changing your mind? None of these responses will warm your heart. They may leave you feeling uncared for and taken for granted. Your preferences

## Attachment: Commitment and Intimacy

don't seem to matter to them. They're not seeing it through your eyes. By the way, this applies even if you're sexually engaged and have a change of heart. It's never too late to say no. It's important to honor your feelings.

Does it make sense that they may be disappointed? Sure. But disappointment doesn't warrant anger, abandonment, or coercion.

Your decision to decline a request for sex doesn't mean it's for a lifetime. It may not even mean that you don't want to spend time with them. You might be happy to hang out with them and be together in a different way.

The challenge here, is for you, the disappointed partner to take a step back, breathe and say something like "You know, I'm disappointed but I know you've been really busy and that you're depleted. Is there another way you'd like to spend time together tonight? A walk? A movie? Or do you just need to get some rest?" Ironically, accepting "no" and responding with grace and understanding is an act of emotional presence and connection. Over time, this kind of response increases the likelihood of more sexual intimacy in your relationship.

> **Exercise: Share Your "Where to Begin" Exploration**
>
> Review your journal entry regarding "where to begin." Share what you want your partner to know and understand. Even though your position impacts them, it's about you and what's right for you to be able to move forward.

While initiating sexual intimacy can be complex, it's especially so in the aftermath of infidelity. Your partner might be clear in communicating a desire for sex or they might be quite indirect. They might make the request with words, a hug, a look or even a complaint. "Don't you ever even think about sex?" Certainly, more personal words like "I miss you" or "I really want to be close to you" are more likely to be well received. However they approach you, it's important that your preferences and your voice matters.

### Exercise: Requesting Sex

Take a moment to explore the issue of initiating sexual intimacy. What feels right? What doesn't? Start with your journal.

- Describe how your partner approaches you for sexual intimacy? Is it via words, personal or impersonal...touch, sexual or affectionate...or an action?

- How does it feel to you? Does it leave you feeling loved, desired, and respected?

- How you would like to be approached. What could they say or do that would feel right to you?

- How do you request sexual intimacy? Is it via words, personal or impersonal ... touch, sexual or affectionate...or an action?

- Do you like to make the request, or would you prefer your partner to do so?

- How would you be most comfortable initiating sex?

- How would your partner like to be approached when you're interested in sex?

### Exercise: Refusing Sex

Take a moment to craft words to use in declining an invitation for sexual intimacy. Enter this in your journal.

If your partner approaches you and you're not in the mood, are you free to say no? What words would you use?

If you approach your partner and they decline your offer, what words would you like to hear?

In this situation, a little grace goes a long way.

> ### Exercise: **Talking About Sexual Touch**
>
> Think about your history of sexual touch with your partner. Revisit it from the early days of your relationship to the present. That "touch history" remains embedded in your nervous system even to this day. Perhaps some was comfortable and connecting. Maybe other moments less so. In the wake of the betrayal, as you look to the future, learning from this history is important.
>
> Revisit your experience of sexual touch with your partner through the following questions. Enter your responses in your journal, then have a conversation when the time is right.
>
> - What types of sexual touch with your partner were most connecting?
> - Were you able to share this with your partner? How did they respond?
> - What kinds of sexual touch just never felt right?
> - Were you able to share this with your partner? How did they respond?
> - When you look to the future, what kind of sexual touch appeals to you?
> - Are there types of sexual touch that have lost their appeal or left you feeling used?

# In Closing

In this chapter, you focused on the pivotal issues of commitment as well as emotional and sexual intimacy. They're essential as you solidify your recovery. They're the challenge of today and the work of a lifetime. Your story started long ago, has been updated today, and calls for time and attention as you move forward.

CHAPTER 11

# Making It Forever

We'll complete the healing journey with attention to preserving and deepening the gains you've made. The focus will be on creating patterns and strategies to keep both of you leaning in. They'll help you stay close and connected. They'll also serve as safeguards against the negative impact of drift and avoidance.

## Protecting Your Progress

Managing life stress is an important relationship skill. The stress being addressed here is not tension about your relationship but the stressors of everyday life. Problems with your boss, coworker gossip, the neighbor's barking dog, broken water pipes, or an unexpected car repair can have a negative effect on your relationship. It's called *spillover stress*, and when you don't manage it well, when you don't manage it together, it creates a crack in your bond (Gottman and Gottman 2024). This single issue has a powerful impact on your ability to maintain the gains you've made and the connection you've created.

Why is this so powerful? Let's return to the idea of your go-to person. While some minor stressors can be handled alone, issues that are chronic or intense are better shared with your loved one. Bringing them to your partner can lighten the load. You don't feel so alone. You feel understood and supported. Is the issue still there? Of course, but it doesn't weigh on you quite so heavily. A positive conversation with your partner gives you something of value. It's a deposit in your *emotional bank account* (Gottman and Gottman 2024). And building this account with small deposits on a regular basis is essential.

There is, however, one caveat. The value of this conversation with your partner is based on the premise that you experience them as attuned, understanding, and supportive. This is a time when presence, interest, and compassion are called for.

And when your partner comes to you with a life stress, being their go-to person doesn't mean you might not have your own thoughts about the issue. You might even feel you can see what your partner is doing wrong or what they could do to remedy the situation. Even if you're right, it's not the time to offer your perspective or your wisdom. That comes later…if desired.

Again, the important point here is for you to have the kind of relationship where you can count on your partner to have your back and be there for you, with you. Use the next exercise to develop this listening skill.

---

### Exercise: **Stress-Reducing Conversation**

Make a list of three or four stressors that are on your mind. Remember, they're about external stressors, not things about your relationship with your partner. Even issues you might have with your kids, your family, or your partner's family might be too personal to be considered external stressors. (Use the Gottman-Rapoport exercise in chapter 7 for those issues.) Your stressor could be about something that happened recently, or it might be related to something looming in the near future. Decide which one you would like to share with your partner. When done well, this exercise offers a connecting blend of catharsis and compassion.

Decide who will talk about their concern first. That person is the Speaker. The other partner will begin as the Listener.

Try starting with each person talking for fifteen minutes about their stressor and related themes. This fifteen-minute suggestion isn't rigid but it sometimes helps to have a shared idea of how much time will be dedicated to the exercise. Both of you need the opportunity to share. If you simply don't have the time for this kind of interaction on a daily basis, adapt it to fit your life. Some couples reduce it to ten minutes each. Others do it two or three times a week. The main caution is that if you don't make these conversations part of your regular life flow, they will dissipate over time.

*Speaker's role.* Simply talk about the issue and how you experience it. Describe the situation. Share your views, thoughts and opinions. Let it out and let them in on what it's like for you. Be sure to share your feelings. Your anger, fear or sadness. Perhaps even hopelessness.

*Listener's role.* As the Listener, your role is to simply be there for your partner. Put your views on the back burner. Put yourself in their shoes and try to understand what they're experiencing, what they're feeling. At times, you might reflect what you're hearing: "So, you're saying, you stepped away from your desk for three minutes to help a coworker and your boss jumped on you in front of the whole office, accusing you of taking an unauthorized break? He didn't even check with you about why you weren't at your desk. Is that right?" If you're having an empathic reaction, you might comment on that too. "I can see why that would be upsetting…even embarrassing. I'm sorry you had to go through that." But generally, keep your focus on your partner.

It's especially important to stay away from defending the person your partner is struggling with. It's called "siding with the enemy," which sabotages the intent of the exercise. Remember, this exercise is about helping your partner feel that you're there with them. To know that they're not alone.

Here are a few questions you might use:

- "Tell me more about how this really started."
- "How did it affect you at first?"
- "What's the most upsetting part of this for you?"
- "What happens inside when you begin to feel overwhelmed?"
- "What are the most painful parts of it?"
- "What's your greatest fear about this? The worst possible outcome?"
- "What can you imagine that would make it better?"
- "What can I do to support you through this?"

> - "What do you need?"
>
> Brief closing comments add a nice punctuation to the process.
>
> Listener: "Thanks for letting me in on that. I like knowing what you're going through and how you're feeling!"
>
> Speaker: "Thanks for taking the time to hear my upset. It helps to share it with you."
>
> End the sharing session with an appreciation, perhaps even a hug...the twenty-second variety.
>
> Now switch roles and be there for your partner as they share an experience of the day.
>
> Practice the stress-reducing conversation, even an abbreviated form of it, on a daily basis.

## Maintaining Connection

Here are some simple ways to keep your love alive.

### Transitions

Look for moments in the pattern of your daily living that set a tone or create a feeling of good will between you. Situations like the shift from sleep to waking, when one of you leaves for work, when you're finally home together after work, and as you prepare for bed are common times to consider. Transition rituals can offer a large payoff for a small amount of time. (See chapter 8.)

### Admiration and Appreciation

This is another opportunity to create moments of connection even when time is limited. Get in the habit of letting your partner know you see and value them. Pay particular attention to who they are: the personal qualities you see and value in them such as their being loving, energetic, thoughtful, fun, attractive, and creative. This is in addition to what they do, such as chores or responsibilities. Make this part of your daily flow. (See chapter 8.)

## Physical Affection

This of course has to be welcomed and not imposed, but the presence of affectionate, nonsexual touch is an important component of a couple's connection. In the wake of an affair, the HP's feelings and preferences must guide the way. Their feelings determine if, what, when, where, and how affectionate touch can become part of the relationship pattern. The twenty-second hug or six-second kiss might eventually become part of the pattern. Remember, affectionate touch is not the same as sexual touch. (See chapter 10.)

## Weekly Date

This is about prioritizing your personal relationship, your romantic relationship. It's more than a break from the mundane; it's a symbol that *I matter to you*. Make it fit your mood. Above all, get it on your calendar. If you just don't have the time, money, or childcare resources to do it weekly, do it less frequently…but regularly. Sticking to a schedule matters. (See chapter 8.)

## State of the Union

Here's a new ritual to consider. The state of the union ritual is a weekly check-in that focuses on your experience of your relationship during the past week (Gottman and Gottman 2024). It protects you from drift, that insidious process that can trigger a cascade of negative moments that erode your bond. This weekly check-in begins with recounting and sharing some positive moments or feelings from the week and ends with an eye toward the coming week and what you need from each other. The central focus of the experience is to counter any tendency toward avoidance by inviting you to talk about issues or concerns that have begun to bubble. Catch emerging issues before they become problems. Talk about them before they take root.

As you enter the "issue" phase of this ritual, prepare yourself to share as well as listen. Commit to hearing your partner's words and giving them the benefit of the doubt. Be mindful of self-regulation and not turning to the Four Horsemen. Remember the processes of accepting influence and repair. Depending on the issue, you might use one of the protocols in chapter 7. This is an opportunity to be sure you don't let the communication muscles you've developed atrophy.

Make this a regular part of your week. Set it up for success. Identify a day and time of day that permits you to bring your best self to the conversation. It doesn't work well when you're depleted. Create a context of peace and privacy, a setting that's calming to you.

---

### Exercise: **State of the Union**

Agree to the time and place for a weekly relationship hour. Arrive rested and in a positive frame of mind.

1. Spend the first few minutes activating your friendship. Share five appreciations you have from the previous week. (This requires a bit of awareness during the week. Noticing positive things about your partner is a great habit to develop.)

2. Now, talk about the issues on your mind. What would you like to discuss first? You might use the Gottman-Rapoport intervention to permit both of you to express how you feel and share a *positive need* about the topic. If there was a fight that's still on your mind, the Aftermath of a Fight or Regrettable Incident exercise may be the right call. Maybe a Dreams Within Conflict or Compromise Ovals exercise fits the issue. Perhaps it's none of these. You might just want to work on friendship. Agree on the focus of this conversation and bring your *best self* to the exchange. End the working

> part of the hour by sharing appreciations for being willing to talk about rather than avoid the issue.
>
> 3. Close with the question "What can I do this week to make you feel loved and appreciated?" Remember to share it as a positive need: what you *do* want rather than something you don't want.

# In Closing

You've done the work to rebuild your bond and put your relationship on solid footing. It's been an intense journey, with moments of heaven and hell sprinkled throughout. You've endured a lot and learned a lot as you have created a path to connection. Now create the time to walk that path together. You're stronger now, both as individuals and as a couple. Your communication skills will serve you well as you move forward. You know how to deal with conflict, build friendship, and dream together once again. Perhaps more importantly, you've come once again to see and appreciate the beauty of the partner you chose long ago and choose again today. Stay close. Stay connected. Stay committed. You have something worth preserving.

# References

Atkins, D. C., D. H. Baucom, and N.S. Jacobson. 2001. "Understanding Infidelity: Correlates in a National Random Sample." *Journal of Family Psychology* 15(4): 735–749.

Badiou, A. 2009. *In Praise of Love.* New York: The New Press.

Bowlby, J. 1982. *Attachment and Loss. Volume 1: Attachment,* 2nd ed. New York: Basic Books.

Cacioppo, J. T., and L. G. Tassinary. *1990 Principles of Psychophysiology: Physical, Social and Inferential Elements.* Cambridge University Press.

Doherty, W. J. 1997. *The Intentional Family.* New York: Harper Collins.

Field, T. 2001. *Touch.* Cambridge, MA: MIT Press.

Frankl, V. E. 1946. *Man's Search for Meaning.* New York: Simon and Schuster.

Glass, S. P., and J.C. Staeheli. 2003. *Not "Just Friends": Protect Your Relationship from Infidelity and Heal the Trauma of Betrayal.* New York: Free Press.

Gottman, J. M. 2011. *The Science of Trust: Emotional Attunement for Couples.* New York: W. W. Norton and Company.

Gottman, J. M., and J. DeClaire. 2001. *The Relationship Cure. A 5 Step Guide for Building Better Connections with Family, Friends and Lovers.* New York: Crown.

Gottman, J. M., J. Driver, and A. Tabares. 2015. "Repair During Marital Conflict in Newlyweds: How Couples Move from Attack-Defend to Collaboration." *Journal of Family Psychotherapy* 26(2): 85–108.

Gottman, J., and J. Gottman. 2017. *Treating Affairs and Trauma: Helping Couples Heal and Rebuild Trust.* The Gottman Institute.

Gottman, J., and J. Gottman. 2018. *The Science of Family and Couples Therapy: Behind the Scenes at the Love Lab.* New York: W. W. Norton and Company.

Gottman, J. M., and J.S. Gottman. 2022. The Love Prescription: Seven Days to More Intimacy, Connection and Joy. New York: Penguin Life Books.

Gottman, J. M., and J.S. Gottman. 2024. *The New Marriage Clinic: A Scientifically Based Marital Therapy.* New York: W. W. Norton and Company. Norton Professional Books.

Gottman, J., S., and J.M. Gottman. 2024. *Fight Right: How Successful Couples Turn Conflict into Connection.* New York: Harmony Books.

Gottman, J. M., J.S. Gottman, D. Abrams, and R.C. Abrams. 2008. *Eight Dates: Essential Conversations for a Lifetime of Love*. New York: Workman Publishing.

Gottman, J. M., L.F. Katz, and C. Hooven. 1997. *Meta-Emotions*. Hillsdale, NJ: Erlbaum.

Gottman, J. M., and N. Silver. 2015. *The Seven Principles for Making Marriage Work: A Practical Guide from the Country's Foremost Relationship Expert*. New York: Harmony Books.

Gottman, J. M., and N. Silver. 2012. *What Makes Love Last? How to Build Trust and Avoid Betrayal*. New York: Simon and Schuster.

Irvine, T. J., and P.R. Peluso. 2022. "An Affair to Remember: A Mixed-Methods Survey Examining Therapists' Experiences Treating Infidelity." *The Family Journal* 30(3): 324–333.

Johnson, S. M. 2013. *Love Sense: The Revolutionary New Science of Romantic Relationships*. New York: Little, Brown and Company.

Lewis, T., F. Amini, and R. Lannon. 2000. *A General Theory of Love*. New York: Vintage Books.

Marano, H. E. 2023. "How to Ask for (and Get) What You Need From Your Partner." *Psychology Today,* November 7. https://www.psychologytoday.com/au/articles/202311/how-to-ask-for-and-get-what-you-need-from-your-partner?msockid=04cf4d6c46c26aca0cf25964476a6b19.

Nagoski, E. 2015. *Come As You Are*. New York: Simon and Schuster.

Northrup, C., P. Schwartz, and J. Witte. 2013. *The Normal Bar: The Surprising Secrets of Happy Couples and What They Reveal About Creating a New Normal in Your Relationship*. 1st ed. New York: Crown Archetype.

Peluso, P. R. 2019. *A Family Systems Guide to Infidelity: Helping Couples Understand, Recover From and Avoid Future Affairs*. London: Routledge.

Robinson, E. A., and M.G. Price. 1980. "Pleasurable Behavior in Relationship Interaction: An Observational Study." *Journal of Consulting and Clinical Psychology* 48: 117-118.

Rusbult, C. E., C. Agnew, and X. Arriaga. 2011. "The Investment Model of Commitment Processes." *Department of Psychological Sciences Faculty Publications*. Paper 26.

Rusbult, C. E., J.M. Martz, and C.R. Agnew. 1998. "The Investment Model Scale: Measuring Commitment Level, Satisfaction Level, Quality of Alternatives, and Investment Size." *Personal Relationships* 5: 357 – 391.

Spring, J. A., and M. Spring. 2022. *How Can I Forgive You? The Courage to Forgive, the Freedom Not To*. 2nd ed. New York: Harper.

**William M. Bumberry, PhD**, is a licensed psychologist with more than twenty-five years' experience treating couples. He is a Certified Gottman Therapist, Consultant, and Senior Trainer. Bumberry has been affiliated with the Gottman Institute for more than two decades. He has conducted more than a hundred Gottman professional trainings nationally and internationally, and is passionate about helping clinicians bring the Gottman Method into their life's work. He is a member of the American Psychological Association. In addition to his expertise in the Gottman Method, Bumberry is certified in emotionally focused therapy (EFT). He is coauthor of *Dancing with the Family* and *Reshaping Family Relationships*. He has a couples-based private practice in St. Louis, MO.

Foreword writer **John Flanagan, AMHSW**, is partner at the Relationship Institute of Australasia, and principal at Burleigh Heads Psychology and Relationship Clinic. He is a mental health–accredited social worker with a masters in Gestalt therapy, and is an Advanced Clinical Trainer and Consultant with the Gottman Institute.

Foreword writer **Trish Purnell-Webb, MPsych(Clin)**, is partner at the Relationship Institute of Australasia. She is a clinical psychologist, Certified Gottman Therapist, Advanced Clinical Trainer, and Consultant for the Gottman Institute.

# Real change *is* possible

For more than fifty years, New Harbinger has published proven-effective self-help books and pioneering workbooks to help readers of all ages and backgrounds improve mental health and well-being, and achieve lasting personal growth. In addition, our spirituality books offer profound guidance for deepening awareness and cultivating healing, self-discovery, and fulfillment.

Founded by psychologist Matthew McKay and Patrick Fanning, New Harbinger is proud to be an independent, employee-owned company. Our books reflect our core values of integrity, innovation, commitment, sustainability, compassion, and trust. Written by leaders in the field and recommended by therapists worldwide, New Harbinger books are practical, accessible, and provide real tools for real change.

**newharbingerpublications**

# MORE BOOKS from NEW HARBINGER PUBLICATIONS

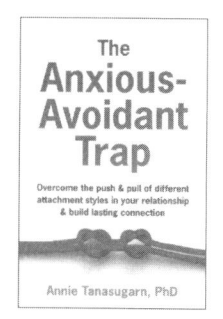

**THE ANXIOUS-AVOIDANT TRAP**
Overcome the Push and Pull of Different Attachment Styles in Your Relationship and Build Lasting Connection
978-1648485459 / US $19.95

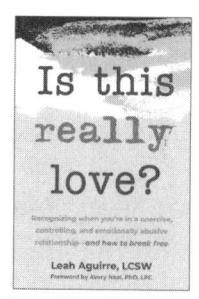

**IS THIS REALLY LOVE?**
Recognizing When You're in a Coercive, Controlling, and Emotionally Abusive Relationship—and How to Break Free
978-1648485480 / US $19.95

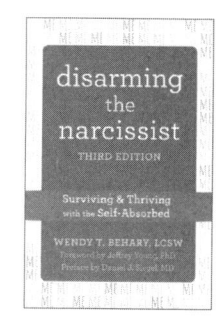

**DISARMING THE NARCISSIST, THIRD EDITION**
Surviving and Thriving with the Self-Absorbed
978-1684037704 / US $19.95

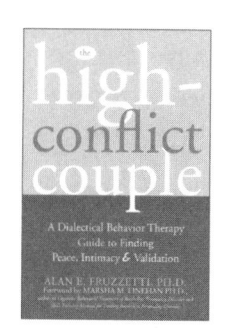

**THE HIGH-CONFLICT COUPLE**
A Dialectical Behavior Therapy Guide to Finding Peace, Intimacy, and Validation
978-1572244504 / US $19.95

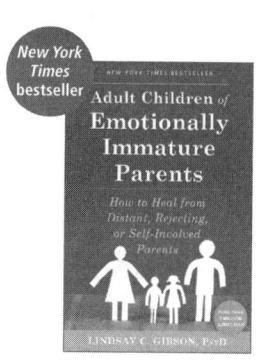

**ADULT CHILDREN OF EMOTIONALLY IMMATURE PARENTS**
How to Heal from Distant, Rejecting, or Self-Involved Parents
978-1626251700 / US $18.95

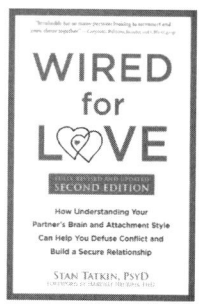

**WIRED FOR LOVE, SECOND EDITION**
How Understanding Your Partner's Brain and Attachment Style Can Help You Defuse Conflict and Build a Secure Relationship
978-1648482960 / US $19.95

**newharbingerpublications**
1-800-748-6273 / newharbinger.com

(VISA, MC, AMEX / prices subject to change without notice)
Follow Us

Don't miss out on new books from New Harbinger.
Subscribe to our email list at **newharbinger.com/subscribe**

# Did you know there are **free tools** you can download for this book?

Free tools are things like **worksheets, guided meditation exercises**, and **more** that will help you get the most out of your book.

You can download free tools for this book—whether you bought or borrowed it, in any format, from any source—from the New Harbinger website. All you need is a NewHarbinger.com account. Just use the URL provided in this book to view the free tools that are available for it. Then, click on the "download" button for the free tool you want, and follow the prompts that appear to log in to your NewHarbinger.com account and download the material.

You can also save the free tools for this book to your **Free Tools Library** so you can access them again anytime, just by logging in to your account! Just look for this button on the book's free tools page.

**+ Save this to my free tools library**

If you need help accessing or downloading free tools, visit **newharbinger.com/faq** or contact us at **customerservice@newharbinger.com**.